Your Home Remedy for Acid Reflux Disease
Live, Eat and Heal Abundantly

Howard Christian Ph.D.

Copyright © 2025 by Howard Christian Ph.D.

All rights reserved. No part of this book may be reproduced in any form without written permission from the publisher or author. Howard Christian Ph.D. asserts the moral right to be identified as the author of this work.

Disclaimer

This book is intended for informational purposes only. It is not a substitute for professional medical advice, diagnosis, or treatment. Always consult a physician or qualified health professional regarding any medical condition. Never disregard professional medical advice or delay seeking help because of something you have read in this book. While this book contains information about emotional, mental, and physical well-being based on the author and others' experiences, the author is not a health professional, and the information is not intended as a substitute for professional medical or psychological advice. If you are experiencing mental health issues, such as depression, anxiety, or suicidal thoughts, consult a qualified mental health professional immediately. Statements in this book have not been evaluated by the U.S. Food and Drug Administration and are not intended to diagnose, treat, cure, or prevent any disease. This book does not provide specific medical or psychological diagnosis or treatment. Individual results may vary, and no guarantees of effectiveness are made. External links within this book may direct readers to third-party websites over which the author and publisher have no control and for which they are not responsible for any information or claims made therein. Readers should exercise discretion in accessing external resources. The author and publisher assume no responsibility for any health consequences resulting from the application or reliance on the information provided. By using this book, you accept full responsibility for your actions and decisions. This book may be updated periodically. While efforts are made to keep content current, the author and publisher make no guarantees regarding the accuracy, completeness or reliability of the information, and they disclaim all warranties. To the fullest extent permitted by applicable law, the author and publisher disclaim all liability for any direct, indirect, incidental, special, consequential, or punitive damages arising from or relating to your use of this book or any information contained herein. The views expressed in this book are those of the author and do not necessarily reflect the opinions of any organizations or institutions the author may be affiliated with. By reading this book, you acknowledge that you have read and understood this disclaimer and agree to accept its terms.

First edition 2025 Your Home Remedy Limited
ISBN: 978-0-9922536-0-8

To my beloved son, Will, whose light will forever illuminate my heart, and to RA, YR, LB, and SL, with whom I share the deep ache of his loss;

And to all who suffer, may you find meaning in your struggle, compassion for yourselves, kindness for others, and comfort within these pages.

"I saw the crescent. You saw the whole of the moon."

— The Waterboys

Contents

Acknowledgments	VII
Author's Note on Terms	IX
Get Connected!	XI
Glossary	XII

I: Why We Need a New Understanding of Disease

1. Dear Reader,	3
2. GERD—the Dualistic Biomedical Perspective	7
3. GERD—Opening to a MindBody Perspective	15
4. Exploring a Meaning-Based Story Approach	25
5. Skepticism is Welcome: Addressing Your Hesitancy	39

II: Disease and Story

6. Symptoms, Story and Meaning	51
7. The Five P's	59
8. The Stomach as Metaphor	67
9. Your Story	77
10. Identifying Specific Memories	85
11. Unearthing the Phenomenon	93
12. Hermes, the Messenger	103
13. Working with Symbols	111

14. Charting Your Symptoms — 125

III: Working with Feelings

    15. Affect, Emotion, Feeling and Communication — 133

    16. We Are Trained Not To Feel — 139

    17. Attuning to Feelings — 153

    18. Giving Feelings a Name — 163

    19. Accepting and Reframing Feelings through Energy Psychology — 171

    20. Feelings as Connection — 187

IV: Generative Healing

    21. Self-Nurturing: Ideas for Filling Your Bucket — 205

    22. Getting Therapeutic Support for GERD — 215

    23. Why Do We Suffer? — 233

    Stay Connected! — 236

Acknowledgments

This book emerged from my own discomfort and the struggles of many brave souls who recognized the value of suffering—and, through empathy, the suffering of others. They applied these lessons with such grace and humility so as to grow and love and share in ways that allowed me to benefit. I stand on the shoulders of these giants.

The first of these is Mrs Buckton, my teacher, who in 1977 taught me that behavioral change comes from the unconditional love we can give to others' unlovely parts. Thanks also to Mrs H. M. Howie and Mr Bob Overend, teachers too, who taught me the value of the words I could express. As a scientist and communicator I benefited from the echo of their relentless encouragement. I continue to benefit now too.

Of course none of what follows would have been possible without Misters Don Johnson, Louis Borok and A. H. Salter. Teachers all, but social workers and humanitarians first. That I am here today is the result of your discreet intervention and tacit encouragement to find a reason.

To Associate Professor Glenn S. "Buck" Buchan, PhD, Professor Margaret Baird, PhD, and Professor John M. B. "Sandy" Smith, PhD, who taught me the practices as well as principles of science, and the means to its integrity. You gave me so much and were all taken, by cancer, too soon. I miss your fellowship and wisdom, but most of all I miss your humanity. You each inspired me to be more creative in the ways we can help others.

To Adjunct Professor Dr. Brian Broom, MBChB, FRACP, MNZAP, who as a consultant immunologist, psychotherapist, MindBody luminary and often "doctor of last resort" has earned the right to insist that "wholeperson" and "MindBody" are written—and practiced—without a hyphen. Your dedication to uplifting others has been instrumental in making this book a reality. I can only encourage others to embrace the wealth of knowledge so artfully shared in your MindBody training program, your lectures, your case presentations, and your books. When I sat in your office in 2006 as a patient, your smorgasbord question gave me the shock of my life. While this shock didn't lead us into a healing conversation, it did precipitate my own passion for philosophy and its promise to one day dismantle humanity's enduring Cartesian crisis. Thank you for being the pathfinder and showing me the value of your aggressive brand of listening. Because of you I am finally in my bodymind and ready to speak.

With Brian as trailblazer and visionary, Josie Goulding, MHSc, DipPsych, DipNursing was my torchbearer and navigator. Your relentless insistence on wanting more for me as a student of MindBody and as a person struggling for wholeness made me a better practitioner and coach, but more importantly set me on a journey to undertake my own personal work. More than one person is grateful to you as a result.

Mark Skelding, DipPsych, MEd, you were the healing guide and ecopsychologist in whose therapeutic practice I found many answers and some important questions besides. Without your fearless presence in my life I would still be stuck, a lesser version of the man I am today. I would not have been accountable when the levees finally broke, but instead waiting on the poorly signed back roads of being. Thank you, eternally, for helping me to create virtuous, self-augmenting ripples in the universal fabric of consciousness to foster courage and the acceptance, healing and belonging we all need.

To Dr. Karen Kent, PhD, and Randal and Karene Scott, my stalwarts, crisis responders, problem solvers and value guardians, I owe so much. Thank you for your unconditional love and divine forbearance. You are each a gift to the world and a gem to me.

To Frances Key Phillips, BA, MPH, my editor, I would like to extend my deep gratitude for your consistent encouragement and laser focus. You have generously and lovingly embraced and nourished the ideas on these pages, giving them the chance to flourish within the hearts and minds of those who have patiently awaited this moment.

Finally, to my spirited brothers, Goose, Sam and Johnnie, I'd like to acknowledge your influence, presence, love and unconditional support in my life.

Author's Note on Terms

Acid reflux versus acid reflux disease

Acid reflux occurs when stomach acid flows back into the esophagus, leading to symptoms such as heartburn, regurgitation and abdominal discomfort. In this context, it is appropriate to refer to any symptoms as "acid reflux." This happens occasionally in most people, especially after large meals or when lying down. It is important to note that most people who experience these occasional acid reflux symptoms will not have acid reflux *disease*, medically known as gastro-esophageal reflux disease or GERD.

Acid reflux disease and GERD are terms given to a more severe, chronic manifestation where acid reflux symptoms occur regularly and are associated with an underlying disease process. This can lead to complications and happens when the lower esophageal sphincter (LES) becomes weakened or relaxes inappropriately, allowing the frequent backflow or reflux of stomach contents.

Whereas both "acid reflux disease" and "GERD" refer to the same condition, "GERD" is the clinical term often used in medical contexts, whereas "acid reflux disease" is commonly used in everyday language.

A more recently described disease variant is laryngopharyngeal reflux (LPR), also known as silent reflux because classic symptoms in the chest are often absent. In LPR, stomach acid flows back into the esophagus and into the larynx and throat.

Not everyone with GERD or LPR has received a formal diagnosis from their doctor; many individuals may relate to the discomfort and symptoms commonly described as "acid reflux symptoms," even if they have not been formally diagnosed. This distinction helps clarify the spectrum of experiences related to these terms.

Given the similar symptoms associated with occasional acid reflux and acid reflux disease/GERD, for the sake of clarity and efficiency it is useful to group the entire spectrum of experiences under a single label. For the purposes of this book, whose well-informed readers are more likely to have been diagnosed with GERD or LPR, or whose symptoms are at a frequency and intensity where they are now considering going to the doctor for a formal diagnosis and possible treatment, it is logical to refer to the disease. By using "GERD" as the label of choice, I acknowledge these nuances while facilitating clearer communication.

For convenience, I include a *Glossary* of terms at the front of the book.

Language conventions

A lot of attention in the book is paid to language. This is because we use language symbolically, as well as literally, to express our stories in ways that are enriched with hidden meaning. By paying close attention to the *exact* language we use to express our stories, it is possible to uncover this hidden meaning, which may guide us to an unexpected understanding of self and disease.

While drafting this book, I began to notice my own unconscious use of language within the text; language that in the context of GERD can be regarded as potentially meaningful. I began to emphasize these words and phrases with the intention that the highlighted text would help to elevate the unconscious aspect of your suffering to its full consciousness. However, it became apparent that this highlighting may be more distracting than helpful. For this reason, I have limited this emphasis to only two chapters: *Symptoms, story and meaning* and *The stomach as metaphor*.

Get Connected!

Your Home Remedy for Acid Reflux Disease

Free Companion Resources

Enhance your journey with *Your Home Remedy for Acid Reflux Disease: Live, Eat and Heal Abundantly* by unlocking a treasure trove of FREE Companion Resources. Dive into symptom-mood charts, exclusive audio exercises, and a transformative MindBody workbook designed to accelerate your healing from acid reflux disease/GERD. And this is just the beginning—stay tuned for more bonus content coming your way!

Don't wait—visit the link below to gain instant access and enhance your journey to wellness today!

HOWARDCHRISTIAN.COM/READER-COMPANION-RESOURCES

Live, Eat and Heal Abundantly

Glossary

Acid reflux: The occasional and normally mild occurrence of stomach acid flowing back into the esophagus, causing temporary discomfort.

Acid reflux disease: A chronic condition in which stomach acid frequently flows back into the esophagus, causing symptoms such as heartburn, regurgitation, and other related symptoms.

Acupressure: A healing technique that involves applying pressure to specific points on the body to relieve symptoms and promote healing.

Acute: Describes a condition or disease characterized by a sudden onset and often severe or intense symptoms that typically have a short duration.

Adaptive: A learned response to an environmental stimulus or stressor that represents a modification or change in a previous response, enabling better adjustment to new conditions.

Affective behavior: Actions, expressions, or responses that are influenced by or related to emotions, feelings, and moods.

Affect (psychology): The underlying experience of emotion or mood, as well as its observable expression, such as through facial expressions, tone of voice, body language, and behaviors.

Affect regulation: The predominantly unconscious process, heavily influenced by early childhood experiences, through which individuals manage their emotions to maintain balance and adapt to their surroundings.

Assumption: A statement or belief that is taken for granted, often serving as a foundation for further reasoning or decision-making.

Attachment disorder: A psychological condition stemming from a lack of healthy emotional bonds with a child's primary caregivers during early childhood, leading to difficulties in forming secure relationships.

Attachment theory: A psychological theory that emphasizes the importance of early emotional bonds formed between a child and their primary caregiver and how these bonds influence emotional and social development throughout life.

Attunement: The ability to recognize one's own emotional state through bodily sensations and to modulate that emotional state to achieve harmony with another person's feelings, facilitating effective connection and understanding.

Biomedical: Refers to the interdisciplinary field that combines biological and medical sciences, operating under a model that recognizes only physical phenomena as the causative agents of disease and focuses treatment on the physical modification of disease signs and symptoms.

Bodymind: A wholeperson representation of personhood in which body and mind are considered to be inseparable when seen through the lens of a MindBody philosophy (see: wholeperson, MindBody).

Chronic: Describes a condition or disease that is long-lasting, persistent, and often progressive, typically lasting for three months or longer and requiring ongoing management or treatment.

Clinical psychology: A branch of psychology focused on the assessment, diagnosis, and treatment of mental disorders and psychological suffering, which has evolved along complementary lines to the biomedical model, prioritizing a physical understanding of psychological reality.

Cognition: The mental processes involved in acquiring, processing, and storing information, including perception, memory, reasoning, problem-solving, and decision-making.

Cognitive-behavioral therapy: Cognitive-behavioral therapy (CBT) is a structured, time-limited psychotherapy that aims to identify and modify negative thought patterns and behaviors, helping individuals develop healthier coping strategies and improve emotional regulation.

Coherence (physiology): A measurable physiological state of harmonious functioning in which physiological systems, such as heart rate variability, respiratory patterns, and brain activity, work in synchrony, contributing to overall health, emotional well-being, and optimal performance.

Consciousness: The state of being aware of and able to think about one's own existence, thoughts, feelings, and environment. Understood as a nonlocal phenomenon from a MindBody perspective, suggesting it exists beyond specific physical locations; from a Western, materialistic perspective, it is seen as a localized phenomenon, tied to brain activity.

Core lament: Refers to a fundamental or deep-seated expression of sorrow, grief, or emotional pain that relates to unresolved issues, loss, or significant life experiences, often influencing a person's emotional state and relationships.

Counseling: A professional guidance process that involves talking with a trained counselor to address personal, social, psychological, or physical challenges, fostering self-awareness, problem-solving, and emotional well-being through supportive conversation and therapeutic techniques.

Defenses (psychology): Unconscious psychological strategies used by individuals to protect themselves from anxiety, emotional pain, or unwanted thoughts, helping to manage feelings and maintain psychological balance.

Dualism: A philosophical perspective that posits the existence of two distinct and separate entities: the mind and the body, suggesting that mental phenomena are not reducible to physical processes and that both aspects interact but remain fundamentally different in nature.

Embodiment: The experience of physiological sensations, emotions, thoughts, memories, language, behaviors, and culture, as expressed and understood through the lived experience of the bodymind as a whole.

Emotion: A complex psychological state that involves a subjective experience, physiological response, and expressive behavior, influencing thoughts and actions in response to internal or external stimuli.

Emotional security: The sense of safety and stability an individual feels when their basic needs are met within the context of their relationships and environment, fostering trust and confidence that allows for open emotional expression without fear.

Esophagus (oesophagus): A muscular tube that connects the throat (pharynx) to the stomach, facilitating the transport of food and liquids through coordinated muscular contractions known as peristalsis.

Existentialism (psychology): A philosophical approach that emphasizes individual existence, freedom, and choice, focusing on the subjective experience of individuals and the inherent meaning or lack thereof in life, while exploring themes such as anxiety, responsibility, and the search for authenticity.

Feeling: The conscious recognition and naming of an emotional experience, which involves cognitive effort to distinguish that emotion from others that arise from similar subjective experiences.

Feminism (psychology): A philosophical approach that examines the ways in which gender influences psychological processes, advocating for the recognition of women's experiences and perspectives, challenging traditional power dynamics, and promoting social justice and equality in mental health and psychological research.

Frame (psychology): A specific context or perspective through which individuals interpret and understand experiences, events, and information, influencing their perceptions, attitudes, and behaviors.

GERD: Gastro-esophageal reflux disease or GERD is the clinical term for acid reflux disease most often used in medical contexts (see: acid reflux disease).

Gestalt (psychology): A philosophical approach that emphasizes the understanding of mental processes as organized wholes rather than individual components, highlighting how people perceive and experience patterns, structures, and relationships in their environment to find meaning.

Heartburn: An often painful burning sensation in the chest or throat caused by the reflux of stomach acid into the esophagus, commonly occurring after eating or when lying down.

Heart rate variability: The variation in time interval between successive heartbeats, indicating the body's ability to respond to stress and regulate autonomic functions, with higher variability associated with better health outcomes.

Hermeneutics: The theory and methodology of interpretation, particularly of texts, symbols, and expressions, focusing on understanding meaning through context, historical background, and the perspectives of both the author of the text and its interpreter.

Holistic: Refers to an approach that considers the whole system, including the interconnectedness of its parts, rather than focusing solely on individual components, often applied in contexts such as health, psychology, and education to emphasize overall well-being (see: wholeperson).

Homunculus: Derived from Latin meaning "little man," the homunculus describes the concept of a whole existing within a part, exemplified in Traditional Chinese Medicine, where the ear is believed to contain representations of all parts of the body, illustrating the idea that smaller structures can embody the entirety of a system.

Humanism (psychology): A philosophical approach that emphasizes the inherent worth and potential of individuals, focusing on personal growth, self-actualization, and the importance of subjective experiences while advocating for a wholeperson understanding of human behavior and the uniqueness of each person.

Intuition: The ability to know something instinctively without the need for conscious reasoning, often characterized by a gut feeling or an immediate insight that arises from accumulated experiences and unconscious processing.

Lifestyle intervention: Specific changes to an individual's daily habits and behaviors, such as diet, exercise, and environmental modifications, to improve overall health and prevent or manage chronic diseases.

Lower esophageal sphincter: The lower esophageal sphincter (LES) is a ring of muscle at the junction of the esophagus and the stomach that functions to prevent the backflow of stomach contents, including acid, into the esophagus, thereby playing a crucial role in digestive health.

Maladaptive: A response or behavior that hinders an individual's ability to adjust effectively to environmental demands or challenges, often leading to negative consequences or dysfunction.

Materialistic (philosophy): The assumption that physical matter is the primary substance of reality, asserting that everything, including thoughts, emotions, and consciousness, can be explained in terms of material interactions and that non-material entities, like the mind, have no independent existence.

Meaning (psychology): Refers to the significance or sense that individuals attribute to their experiences, thoughts, and emotions, influencing their perceptions, behaviors, and overall understanding of life, often explored in contexts such as existential psychology and the search for purpose.

MindBody: Refers to a practical healing philosophy that emphasizes the unity of mental and physical processes, suggesting that psychological and physiological states co-emerge as essential facets of human experience, rather than integrate as two distinct forms.

Mindfulness: The practice of maintaining conscious awareness of the present moment, including bodily sensations, emotions, and thoughts, without judgment, fostering a deeper understanding of one's experiences and promoting mental clarity and emotional well-being.

Mirror neuron: A special class of brain cell that activates both when an individual performs an action and when they observe the same action performed by others, providing a neural basis for understanding social behavior, empathy, and learning through imitation.

Mood: A pervasive and sustained emotional state that influences an individual's perspective and behavior over an extended period, often characterized by feelings such as happiness, sadness, anger, or anxiety, and can be affected by various internal and external factors.

Omeprazole: A medication belonging to the class of proton pump inhibitors used to reduce stomach acid production, commonly prescribed for conditions such as gastroesophageal reflux disease (GERD), and peptic ulcers.

Phenomenon: An event or occurrence that is discoverable through observation and endeavor, often described as remarkable or extraordinary within a specific context, distinguishing between the observable aspects and the underlying reality that can be explored and understood.

Phenomenology: A philosophical approach that explores the study of consciousness and experience, emphasizing the underlying hiddenness of true phenomena and aiming to reveal the essence of these experiences as they are perceived by individuals, often uncovering deeper meanings that may not be immediately visible.

Philosophy: The systematic study of fundamental questions regarding existence, knowledge, values, reason, mind, body, and language, employing critical thinking and analysis to explore and understand the nature of reality and our place within it.

Physical treatment: Therapeutic interventions aimed at enhancing physical health by addressing signs and symptoms rather than underlying causes.

Postmodernism (psychology): An approach that critiques and deconstructs traditional theories and narratives, emphasizing the subjective nature of knowledge, the influence of cultural and social contexts on human behavior, and the fluidity of identity, advocating for diverse perspectives and interpretations in understanding psychological experiences.

Proton pump inhibitor: A class of medications that reduce stomach acid production by blocking the proton pump in the stomach's lining.

Psychodynamic: A psychological perspective that emphasizes the influence of unconscious processes, childhood experiences, and internal conflicts on behavior and mental states, focusing on how these factors shape an individual's emotions, thoughts, and relationships.

Psychotherapy: A formal therapeutic process involving a trained mental health professional and a client, aimed at addressing emotional, psychological, behavioral, or physical issues through various techniques and approaches, such as talk therapy, cognitive-behavioral therapy, psychodynamic therapy, or Mind-Body therapy to enhance well-being and facilitate personal growth.

Regurgitation: The expulsion of undigested stomach contents back into the throat or mouth, often occurring without nausea or the forceful act of vomiting, and can be associated with various gastrointestinal conditions.

Relational mirror: The concept in psychology where an individual's self-perception and understanding of their emotions, behaviors, and identity are reflected and influenced by their interactions and relationships with others, highlighting the importance of social contexts in shaping personal development and self-awareness.

Relational psychotherapy: A therapeutic approach that emphasizes the importance of the therapist-client relationship and the influence of interpersonal dynamics on emotional well-being, focusing on how relationships shape individual experiences and using the therapeutic alliance as a tool for healing and personal growth.

Self-agency: Refers to the capacity of an individual to act independently, make choices, and influence their own life and circumstances, emphasizing personal control, responsibility, and the ability to initiate and direct one's actions and decisions.

Shaman: A healer found in various cultures, who is believed to have the ability to communicate with the spirit world, perform rituals, and access altered states of consciousness for healing, guidance, and the integration of spiritual and physical aspects of life.

Sign (medicine): An objective indicator of a medical condition, observable by a healthcare professional during an examination, such as a rash, elevated temperature, or abnormal heart sounds, which can assist in diagnosing and understanding a patient's health status.

Smorgasbord question: The concept introduced by Brian Broom, referring to a type of inquiry that encompasses diverse and varied responses, used in healthcare to encourage exploration and discussion of patients' concerns, preferences, and experiences in a more comprehensive and patient-centered manner.

Somatic metaphor: The use of bodily experiences and sensations to symbolize or express emotional and psychological states, which emphasizes the unity of physical and psychological experiences.

Spontaneous healing: The unexpected and often unexplainable restoration of health or alleviation of symptoms without formal medical intervention, typically attributed to the body's natural healing processes or changes in mindset and environment.

Stream-of-consciousness: A narrative technique that captures the continuous flow of thoughts, feelings, and associations in an unstructured and often nonlinear manner.

Stressor: Any external or internal event, condition, or stimulus that triggers a stress response in an individual, potentially leading to emotional, physical, or psychological strain or discomfort.

Subjective experience: The personal, internal perception and interpretation of events, emotions, and sensations, shaped by an individual's feelings, thoughts, beliefs, and context, and often differing from objective reality or external observations.

Subjective units of distress: A self-reported scale used to measure an individual's perceived level of distress or discomfort regarding a specific situation or emotional state.

Subjectivity: The quality of being based on or influenced by personal feelings, experiences, and perspectives, emphasizing the individual nature of perception and understanding that varies between people, rather than being solely objective or universal.

Supervision (psychology): A formal process in which one professional provides guidance, support, and feedback to another practitioner, ensuring the quality of clinical practice, fostering professional development, and promoting ethical standards within therapeutic and research contexts.

Symbol: A sign, object, or representation that signifies something else, often conveying complex ideas or concepts through association or meaning that extends beyond its literal interpretation.

Symptom: A subjective indication of a disease or condition reported by the patient, which is perceived as an abnormal experience or change in bodily function, often used alongside objective signs to aid in diagnosis and treatment.

Systems (psychology): A philosophical approach that emphasizes the interconnected and interdependent components within a larger framework, such as families, groups, or organizations, emphasizing how individual behaviors and mental processes are influenced by and contribute to the dynamics of the whole system, often studied within the context of systems theory or ecological models.

Synchronicity: The concept introduced by Carl Jung in which two or more seemingly unrelated, meaningful events happen simultaneously, suggesting an underlying connection that transcends conventional explanations.

Talk therapy: A form of psychotherapy that involves verbal communication between a therapist and a client, aimed at exploring feelings, thoughts, and behaviors to promote psychological and physical healing, self-awareness, and personal growth through various therapeutic methods and techniques.

Trauma: An emotional, psychological and physiological response to an event or series of events that is distressing, harmful, or life-threatening, leading to lasting effects on an individual's mental and physical health, behaviors, and overall functioning; all trauma involves a disruption in the individual's sense of connection to themselves, others, or the world around them.

Unconscious: The aspect of mind involving emotions, thoughts, memories, and desires that are not currently in conscious awareness, influencing behavior and experiences without the individual's direct knowledge or control, often explored in psychology to understand underlying motivations and conflicts.

Unitary: The state of being one or unified, characterized by the absence of divisions or separations, often used to describe concepts, systems, or phenomena that function as a cohesive whole, rather than as individual or distinct parts.

Wholeperson: A philosophical reference to the complete individual, encompassing physical, emotional, mental, social, and spiritual aspects, emphasizing the entirety of these dimensions in understanding health, well-being, and personal development.

Part I: Why We Need a New Understanding of Disease

"We have severed mind and body from story and disease. In Western culture, this severance is several centuries underway and the cost to individual and community health is enormous."

— Dr. Brian Broom, MindBody luminary

ONE

Dear Reader,

Thank you—and thank yourself. By purchasing **Your Home Remedy for Acid Reflux Disease: Live, Eat and Heal Abundantly**, you have not only placed your trust in me but, more importantly, you have turned up for yourself in a big way!

Whether you're seeking information for yourself or a loved one, understanding acid reflux disease—medically termed gastro-esophageal reflux disease (GERD[1])—is the first step toward finding relief. The *acid* in acid reflux disease refers to our stomach acid, which can cause distressing symptoms such as heartburn, regurgitation and abdominal discomfort when it is able to flow or *reflux* into the esophagus. When someone experiences regular and/or more intense symptoms, this may indicate underlying *disease*. When disease is present, it is because there is weakness or inappropriate relaxation of the muscle separating the stomach and esophagus whose role it is to keep stomach acid from flowing into the esophagus.

The intention of this self-help guide is to show you how to heal acid reflux disease (hereafter referred to as GERD). And by *heal*, I don't just mean in the book's subtitle. I am talking about a complete resolution of your symptoms and with it the freedom to live and eat abundantly. Added benefits may include a growing feeling of aliveness and a deeper connection with yourself and those around you.

As a former biomedical scientist, I understand that these statements may cause considerable resistance for some people, especially those with a more skeptical bent. It is natural that anyone new to the practical and surprisingly effortless approach to well-being that I advocate will have questions and concerns. Starting with the chapters *GERD—the dualistic biomedical perspective*, *GERD—opening to a MindBody perspective* and *Exploring a meaning-based story approach*, this book addresses many of these concerns.

As a self-help guide, this book shows you how to connect with your innate capacity for self-healing. If you want to be empowered through this ability to understand and work on your health yourself, ***Your Home Remedy for Acid Reflux Disease: Live, Eat and Heal Abundantly*** will be instrumental to that journey. To see if the moment is right for you to step into a wholeperson approach that addresses your health issues, ask if you recognize yourself in any one of these people:

- I am new to my struggle with GERD and seeking direction, or I have extensive experience but still struggle with daily symptoms.

- I want to reduce dependence on GERD medications while maintaining current treatments, and I am concerned about side effects.

- I have tried conventional treatments, dietary changes, or lifestyle modifications without satisfactory results.

- I seek to understand the root causes of my GERD rather than just managing its symptoms, and I want to find meaning to support my well-being journey.

I have written this book with you in mind, wherever you are in your journey to heal from the strictures GERD places on you and your choices. When I healed my GERD in 2008, I did so through uncovering its **meaning**. This meaning was unique to me and did not come about by following a prescriptive path.

I am not going to present you with prescriptive advice, as that is for your doctor. And if you choose to follow a dietary plan or another lifestyle intervention while working through this book, then good for you. It is important to continue following your intuition; this is integral to healing your GERD and has guided you on your journey thus far. The unique approach that I do offer will draw you toward a deep understanding of personal meaning, empowering you to chart your own course to an abundant life free of GERD and other illnesses you may be struggling with. The one hundred percent natural remedy you will learn does not require you to change your lifestyle or give up eating the foods you love. But you will have to change your perspective on several health-related ideas that have persisted for generations to everyone's detriment.

> **Your Home Remedy for Acid Reflux Disease: Live, Eat and Heal Abundantly** is intended as a journey that you can undertake in your own space and at your own pace. As for any book, you can take breaks—even extended ones—before returning to the journey whenever you are ready. A lot of your healing will occur during your breaks from the book and will result from fresh insights about your disease, as well as increased self-knowledge and intuition, which are natural elements of any healing journey.

Healing GERD and other Illnesses

When I write about healing GERD, I do so from *actual* experience. I come from a place of humility, having experienced the pain of GERD as well as a constellation of other illnesses and their symptoms, which kept me alternately powerless, in pain, and trapped. My career had me focused on being the objectively-informed "expert" in my chosen fields of immunology and biomedicine, a stance which left me all the more confused and frustrated as my suffering—and that of those around me—increased without abatement. Writing this book is my way of sharing what I now know and helping others to understand the meaningful basis of their own illnesses—whether physical or psychological—so they can find healing too.

It is my sincere belief that immersing yourself in this book's accessible ideas will help you to achieve the same healing from GERD and other serious illnesses as I have. It is a journey of profound personal growth that bridges the physical, mental and emotional domains of our experience. It is a journey to wholeness. As you embark on your own transformative path, know that your innate resilience and determination to achieve a healthier, more fulfilling life informs each step toward healing and empowerment.

> I will teach you to journey more consciously with your GERD and begin to unpack its meaningful connections with your story. This meaning-based story approach is the same approach that I used in 2008 to heal my own GERD, and live and eat more abundantly.

---

1. GERD is also known as gastro-oesophageal reflux disease (GORD) in Australia, Ireland, New Zealand and the United Kingdom.

Two

GERD—the Dualistic Biomedical Perspective

> For an introduction to acid reflux and an explanation of terms such as "acid reflux disease" and "GERD," please refer to the *Author's note on terms*, as well as the *Glossary*.

How biomedicine sees GERD

Most people experience mild reflux symptoms on occasion. However, the fact that you are reading this book suggests you or someone you love has bothersome, ongoing reflux symptoms, and may have been diagnosed with GERD.

The influential, dualistic "mind separate from body" biomedical perspective regards GERD as a chronic, persistent medical illness requiring ongoing treatment to manage symptoms. A GERD diagnosis is typically made when someone experiences mild acid reflux symptoms at least twice a week, or moderate-to-severe symptoms at least once per week. GERD can lead to complications like inflammation of the esophagus (esophagitis), a pre-cancerous condition called Barrett's esophagus, and esophageal cancer. Other potential complications include narrowing or tightening of the esophagus, asthma, and dental problems such as gum disease and tooth erosion.

For a person to experience the significant and frequent symptoms associated with GERD, there is an underlying disease process involving the lower esophageal sphincter (LES). Normally, this narrow muscle band separates the stomach from the esophagus. In people with GERD, however, the LES relaxes inappropriately, allowing stomach acid to flow back up into the esophagus and sometimes as far as the mouth. This acid reflux irritates the esophagus and leads to classic symptoms of heartburn, regurgitation and chest pain.

In addition to classic symptoms, GERD sufferers may also experience difficulty swallowing (dysphagia), the sensation of a lump in the throat (globus sensation), nighttime symptoms of cough and disrupted sleep, and new or worsening asthma. Other symptoms include abdominal pain (dyspepsia), bloating, belching, laryngitis, tooth erosion, and bad breath (halitosis). However, only your doctor can diagnose GERD and if you have not already received a diagnosis, it might be a good idea to arrange a visit. The current medical perspective holds that the anatomical changes to the LES associated with GERD are irreversible and necessitate treatment, including with prescription medications, lifestyle changes such as to diet, and possible surgical intervention in particularly severe cases.

> **This self-help guide does not replace the care you receive from your doctor. If you have a new illness or condition, if you have not yet been diagnosed with GERD by a doctor, of if you have not had your symptoms examined and investigated, do not rely exclusively on the information in this book in lieu of seeking medical help.**

As well as running some tests, your doctor may place you on a trial period with a prescription drug, such as a proton pump inhibitor (PPI) or histamine type 2 receptor antagonist (H2RA). PPIs work by blocking the production of stomach acid, whereas H2RAs block the action of histamine, a chemical required for stomach acid production. These drugs can be effective at treating the symptoms of GERD, providing temporary relief from your discomfort. While it is true that all drugs have possible side effects, both of these drug classes are considered to be generally safe for long-term use, if not always effective. If you have any concerns, these are best discussed with your doctor.

Many people try to manage the discomfort of GERD with over-the-counter medications. Although these may be effective in some cases, it is common for people with GERD to need prescription-only medications to better manage their symptoms. So, if you are experiencing frequent or severe GERD symptoms, or are taking over-the-counter medications more than twice a week, please go and see your doctor. I encourage you to get a medical diagnosis and appropriate treatment before using the methods in this book to work towards healing your GERD. In this way, you will continue to receive symptomatic relief while you address the root cause of your disease.

Who gets GERD—and why? Epidemiology and risk

Globally, the number of individuals suffering from GERD and seeking treatment is increasing. Proton pump inhibitors rank among the most widely used medications worldwide. In some regions, GERD has become so prevalent that it is perceived as a cultural norm.[1] The symptoms of GERD are synonymous with indulgence and have such influence on our lives that a thriving industry has grown around various over-the-counter products, as well as prescription medications. We are bombarded with media messages encouraging the use of these quick fixes so we can go about our normal business.

The ignorance of the problem hides a more painful reality, which is that GERD is not a benign illness but a serious and often under-diagnosed disease with a significant impact on quality of life. In 2019, there were an estimated 784 million people living with GERD globally, an increase of almost 80% compared with three decades earlier.[2]

In the US, GERD affects an estimated 18% to 28% of the population, nearly 40% of whom experience persistent symptoms despite ongoing medical treatment. These hard-to-treat patients incur an average of $10,000 more in healthcare costs each year compared with those with more mild GERD symptoms.[3]

Family or genetic factors do have some role in people developing GERD and GERD-related disorders.[4] However, anyone can develop the disease and GERD is one of the most prevalent pathologies doctors see in primary care practice.[5] Although more common in people over age 40, infants and young children can also experience GERD. Today, hospitalizations for GERD including among children are more common now than ever before, and so too are downstream complications of the disease. In particular, Barrett's esophagus and esophageal cancer appear to be increasing over time.[6]

You may well ask, why is the global prevalence of GERD increasing? The medical research offers a number of possible, inter-related explanations:

The population is getting older

Globally, age-standardized rates of GERD are highest in the US, Italy, New Zealand, northern Latin America, the Caribbean, north Africa, the Middle East, and eastern Europe. Rates are lower in high-income Asia Pacific, east Asia, and some countries in western Europe. When standardized for age, GERD trends appear to be stable, leading epidemiologists to attribute the increased GERD prevalence over time to population growth and an aging population.

However, age does not explain the increasing prevalence in high-income North America or in high-income Asia-Pacific where rates are lower than North America but nevertheless increasing over time.[7] Other factors such as body weight, smoking and alcohol consumption are also not useful in explaining the increasing GERD prevalence in certain regions.

Even if it could be shown that age is a universal factor in increasing GERD prevalence, any such explanation is based on the assumption that disease is an inevitable part of aging, yet many older people enjoy remarkable health and are free of disease.

Obesity is on the rise

In the same way that an aging population might result in more GERD-affected individuals, a population with more individuals with obesity—an accepted risk factor for GERD—will also be associated with more individuals having GERD. But this time, younger people are also affected, yet only modest associations have been found between GERD and people with obesity.[8]

Furthermore, the assumption that GERD prevalence relates to obesity prevalence does not explain why normal weight people and non-obese, overweight people can develop GERD as well.

Lifestyle assumptions

With the exception of smoking which has shown decreased participation in recent years,[9] the consumption of alcohol[10] and coffee,[11] and eating a diet high in fat[12]—all reasons given for the increasing GERD prevalence—are significant, albeit unevenly distributed, lifestyle factors in the global population.

Yet, the data relating to lifestyle factors and their associated risk with GERD are often conflicting. Certain trigger foods, including coffee for example, are frequently reported to worsen reflux symptoms, but hard evidence linking consumption to GERD is lacking.[13]

Lifestyle assumptions fail to explain the increasing prevalence of GERD in children and people without contributing lifestyle factors.[14]

Current explanations of GERD are not enough

Despite the abundance of research and speculation, the above explanations are inadequate to guide our understanding of *why* GERD prevalence is increasing in the global population.

Acknowledging the limitations of the biomedical perspective, which takes a population-based approach toward understanding GERD, *individuals* living with the disease will nevertheless have their own unique experiences that may well include established risk factors such as those discussed above. Other risk factors include hiatal hernia, having a connective tissue disorder such as scleroderma, and pregnancy. You may have some or none of these risk factors. GERD symptoms have also been associated with the use of certain drug classes. If you think a drug you are taking is making your symptoms worse, please see your doctor for advice.

Dietary triggers

Certain lifestyle choices and the consumption of a diet rich in recognized trigger foods may worsen your GERD symptoms. It is not surprising then that healthcare practitioners and many GERD sufferers will often recommend a host of lifestyle suggestions for improving symptoms. These include smoking cessation, eating smaller meals, avoiding foods and drinks that trigger symptoms, remaining upright for a period after each meal, elevating the head of your bed, and avoiding tight-fitting clothing.

Many different dietary triggers have been identified, including no doubt some of your favorite foods. It is not my intention to include an exhaustive list of trigger foods here since there are many GERD-specific cookbooks available that are dedicated to providing symptomatic relief based on dietary restriction. However, it is worthwhile emphasizing that certain trigger foods are more frequently reported than others to worsen GERD symptoms, especially fried and spicy foods, red sauces, citrus, chocolate, onion, garlic, coffee, some teas, carbonated drinks, and alcohol.[15]

> The one hundred percent natural remedy that I present has nothing to do with these lifestyle interventions. Instead, you will learn a non-dietary, non-dualistic, lifestyle-affirming "MindBody" or meaning-based story approach to healing your GERD that will allow you to live abundantly and keep eating the foods you love.

GERD is more than just a digestive disease

Where biomedicine is starting to gain ground is in its more recent recognition that GERD may be more than just a digestive disease. A growing body of studies reveals that GERD—along with the functional gastrointestinal disorders like irritable bowel syndrome and functional dyspepsia—is closely linked to the autonomic nervous system (ANS), which regulates involuntary bodily functions like breathing, heart rate, and digestion. These studies indicate that imbalances between the sympathetic nervous system—responsible for the body's response to stress—and the parasympathetic nervous system—which promotes rest and digestion—could play a significant role in your symptoms.[16,17]

A critical measure of autonomic nervous activity is heart rate variability (HRV). HRV refers to the variation in time between heartbeats, which reflects the balance between a person's stress (the sympathetic response) and their relaxation (the parasympathetic response). A person who is more relaxed will show higher HRV than will a person who is stressed. When our autonomic balance is disrupted, as is now being shown in people with GERD, low HRV is correlated with worsening symptoms.

Understanding the imbalance between the body's sympathetic and parasympathetic systems in GERD is important. It points to the need for a broader view through which to understand a person's GERD and how to more effectively heal it, rather than solely relying on medications that target physical symptoms.

However, where biomedicine now sees an opportunity for better GERD *symptom control*—such as through stress management, relaxation techniques and lifestyle adjustments—I see the opportunity for a unique approach that heals the underlying emotional, psychological *and* physical aspects of your GERD. We therefore need to take a fresh look at what actually causes GERD and how we might benefit from this understanding. Beginning with *GERD—opening to a MindBody perspective* this book will give GERD the fresh perspective it needs.

---

1. Nehra, A. K., Alexander, J. A., Loftus, C. G., & Nehra, V., (2018). Proton pump inhibitors: Review of emerging concerns. *Mayo Clinic Proceedings*, 93(2): 240-246.

2. Zhang, D., Liu, S., Li, Z., & Wang, R., (2022). Global, regional and national burden of gastroesophageal reflux disease, 1990-2019: Update from the GBD 2019 study. *Annals of Medicine*, 54(1): 1372-1384.

3. Howden, C.W., Manuel, M., Taylor, D., Jariwala-Parikh, K., & Tkacz, J., (2021). Estimate of refractory reflux disease in the United States: Economic burden and associated clinical characteristics. *Journal of Clinical Gastroenterology*, 55(10): 842-850.

4. Bohmer, A.C., & Schumacher, J., (2017). Insights into the genetics of gastroesophageal reflux disease (GERD) and GERD-related disorders. *Neurogastroenterology & Motility*, 29(2): doi: 10.1111/nmo.13017.

5. Kazakova, T., Danoff, R., Esteva, I., & Shchurin, A., (2023). Gastro-esophageal reflux disease in primary care practice: A narrative review. *Annals of Esophagus*, 6 (June 25).

6. Kellerman, R., & Kintanar, T., (2017). Gastroesophageal reflux disease. *Primary Care*, 44(4): 561-573.

7. GBD 2017 Gastro-oesophageal Reflux Disease Collaborators, (2020). The global, regional, and national burden of gastro-oesophageal reflux disease in 195 countries and territories, 1990–2017: A systematic analysis for the Global Burden of Disease Study 2017. *The Lancet Gastroenterology & Hepatology*, 5: 561-581.

8. Eusebi, L. H., Ratnakumaran, R., Yuan, Y., Solaymani-Dodaran, M., Bazzoli, F., & Ford, A. C., (2018). Global prevalence of, and risk factors for, gastro-oesophageal reflux symptoms: A meta-analysis. *Gut*, 67(3): 430-440.

9. GBD 2015 Tobacco Collaborators, (2017). Smoking prevalence and attributable disease burden in 195 countries and territories, 1990-2015: A systematic analysis from the Global Burden of Disease Study 2015. *Lancet*, 389(10082): 1885-1906.

10. GBD 2019 Risk Factors Collaborators, (2020). Global burden of 87 risk factors in 204 countries and territories, 1990-2019: A systematic analysis for the Global Burden of Disease Study 2019. *Lancet*, 396(10258): 1223-1249.

11. Quadra, G. R., Paranaíba, J. R., Vilas-Boas, J., Roland, F., Amado, A. M., Barros, N., Dias, R. J. P., & Cardoso, S. J., (2020). A global trend of caffeine consumption over time and related environmental impacts. *Environmental Pollution*, 256: 113343.

12. Fox, M., & Prakash Gyawali, C., (2023). Dietary factors involved in GERD management. *Best Practice & Research Clinical Gastroenterology*, Feb-Mar: 62-63.

13. Nehlig, A., (2022). Effects of coffee on the gastro-intestinal tract: A narrative review and literature update. *Nutrients*, 14(2): 399.

14. Friedman, C., Sarantos, G., Katz, S., & Geisler, S., (2021). Understanding gastroesophageal reflux disease in children. *Journal of the American Academy of Physicians Assistants*, 34(2): 12-18.

15. Fox, M., & Prakash Gyawali, C., (2023). Dietary factors involved in GERD management. *Best Practice & Research Clinical Gastroenterology*, Feb-Mar: 62-63.

16. Ali, M. K., & Chen, J. D. Z., (2023). Roles of heart rate variability in assessing autonomic nervous system in functional gastrointestinal disorders: A systematic review. *Diagnostics (Basel)*, 13(2): 293.

17. Milovanovic, B., Filipovic, B., Mitavdzin, S., Zdravkovic, M., Gligorijevic, T., Paunovic, J., & Arsic, M., (2015). Cardiac autonomic dysfunction in patients with gastroesophageal reflux disease. *World Journal of Gastroenterology*, 21(22): 6982-6989.

THREE

GERD—Opening to a MindBody Perspective

Uncovering personal meaning

As you embark on your healing journey, I'd like to warmly welcome you to a space of renewed understanding and personal empowerment. This chapter invites you to reset your beliefs about GERD, allowing you to affirm the intuition you likely have that your suffering has important personal meaning for you, which is yet to be uncovered. Together, we will explore a fresh, non-dualistic "MindBody" perspective whose ultimate aim is to nurture your experience of wholeness, and pave the way for a healthier, happier life.

The MindBody perspective I refer to is about making connections between the *subjective* aspects of your story and your GERD symptoms. When we think about subjectivity, it describes our own uniqueness, the ways in which we know ourselves and our experiences. Because no two people—and no two people's diseases—are the same, exploring this inner subjectivity means that we can approach our disease from our own unique vantage point. When you recognize the connections between your subjective story and symptoms, you can uncover deeper, personal meaning that facilitates healing.[1]

The reason why we need a non-dualistic perspective is that the people we contemporarily rely upon for our healing—doctors—are trained only to look for and see our signs and symptoms (the body part of dualism). A global industry has been built around the evidence-based research, diagnosis, measurement, and treatment of this physical aspect of our suffering. On the other hand, doctors ignore the subjective aspects of our story and suffering due to their training (the mind part of dualism). There is no similar industry built around the self-practice-based evidence of our inner subjectivity. Unfortunately, what doctors cannot see they also cannot attend to. And without being able to see *both* a person's story *and* their symptoms in the same "space" (i.e., the "bodymind" of the wholeperson) there can be no connections which form the vital link to healing and wholeness.

We will explore this inner subjectivity and its connections in ways that you can apply to your own unique story. This MindBody approach—hereafter referred to as a **meaning-based story approach**—is founded on a non-dualistic understanding of reality in which mind and body are not treated as separate compartments, but rather are seen as being inseparable aspects or domains of the wholeperson.

This is the same approach that I used to heal GERD and other illnesses besides. It wasn't always easy: I had to acquire knowledge to gain certain insights, and an important growth edge for me involved developing my creativity and imagination, two things we have in abundance as children, but unlearn as we become more self-critical and skeptical as adults.

> *"Imagination is everything. It is the key to coming attractions."*
>
> — Albert Einstein

I'd like to take pains to let you know that, first and foremost, your self-kindness will enrich your own journey. So too will your creativity and imagination. Remember this if things ever get a little tough. You've come this far, you're ready, you've got what it takes. And the journey is totally worth your effort!

GERD is not the enemy

Because we live in a world of contradictions, I venture the opinion that the more we believe we need to be "fixed", then the more we resist our efforts to be fixed. The quality that underlies this need for fixing is often hedged in guilt and shame.

While these feelings have their uses, they are also powerful antagonists to our healing that must be addressed along our journeys (see: *Working with feelings*).

It is imperative that we stop seeing our disease as the enemy. It is not. There are no enemies here. In the same way that a meaning-based story approach to well-being can work together with the dualistic "mind separate from body" biomedical perspective of healthcare,[2] so too can you learn to embrace your disease. It is not a case of me or my disease, with one claiming victory over the other. A more helpful and measured approach is to regard your disease with a sense of curious detachment, an open awareness that does not require you to pit one idea or state of thinking against another in the name of "curing" or "fixing" your disease.

When we do see GERD as the enemy, all we are ever going to recognize are its symptoms. This is because we have been conditioned over our lifetime to see symptoms as something to control, diminish, suppress, medicate, or fix. And all our disease will ever give us in return is resistance, persistence, defiance, and brokenness. This is the opposite of detachment: It is a fear-based attachment that only has one victor, and in this paradigm the disease always wins.

But when we open to the idea of GERD being a messenger for personal meaning that enables us to experience ourselves in a different way, then we take an important step in bridging the connections between our symptoms and story. So don't shoot the messenger!

Accepting your journey in whatever its form requires being open to vulnerability. Being vulnerable is not weakness, but instead a form of openness we all need if we are to take strength from our stride. If vulnerability is a problem for you—men, be honest with yourselves here—I recommend watching two of the most viewed TEDx talks of all time given by Brené Brown.[3,4]

Challenges, risks and rewards

As for any fresh exploration, you may be concerned about possible risks in following the ideas presented herein. The reality is that the increased self-awareness that accompanies a meaning-based story approach to healing brings enormous benefits in physical and psychosocial well-being, self-agency, relationships, motivation, and purpose. But self-awareness is a two-edged sword that also brings potential downsides or risks. These risks include depression, worsening physical symptoms, and shifting dynamics in your important relationships.

Depression

Depression may arise as you shift the emphasis of your experience of GERD away from its physical symptoms toward the underlying issues that inform your story. As part of healing my GERD, along with resolving the physical symptoms, I experienced a purging of intense feelings that I had been holding onto. For me, this was invigorating. But I also understand that the release of strong feelings can cause considerable discomfort for some people.

This self-help book is geared to help you work through any accompanying feelings, including depression. My own and many other people's experiences of following a meaning-based story approach are that as our physical symptoms improve, any significant feelings are also supported.

> **IMPORTANT: If you become significantly depressed or you believe that your existing depression is worsening, or you have suicidal thoughts, tell someone then seek immediate help from an appropriately qualified health professional.**

Worsening physical symptoms

As with any serious illness, your GERD symptoms are best monitored and managed by your doctor. As I have taken care to explain, this self-help book is not intended to replace medical care. Seeking help from an appropriately qualified medical professional does not hinder you in any way from using this book with the intention of healing your GERD.

This process does not require you to think and act using an either/or approach. Rather, one approach complements the other until you experience complete healing of your disease.

I have found that the best time to work on a disease is when symptoms are flaring. This is when we are motivated to achieve a shift, and when our disease has our full attention. Overall, my own and other people's experiences are that symptoms do not become any worse than at their peak before we start working with our stories.

Relationships

Relationships are right at the heart of our lives. As you embark on your self-healing journey, doubtless you will discover important feelings that have implications for different relationships. This is the true nature of personal growth and is a healthy consequence of the changes we are prepared to make for ourselves.

As I later explain in depth, GERD symptoms often reflect relationship patterns and struggles of which we have been unaware. It is possible that in going deeply into your story, you might feel that you need to choose between better health and having stability in your relationships.

If this begins to feel true for you, it is a further example of the either/or thinking that can narrow our possibilities in life: Either I can enjoy better health but my relationships will suffer; or I will have to live with my GERD but at least my relationships remain the same.

The reality is that your physical GERD symptoms can be a consequence of you burying or swallowing uncomfortable feelings that might otherwise create conflict in certain relationships. Addressing these feelings is key to your personal growth. With this shift in perspective, you now have expanded options: I can have better physical health AND improved interpersonal relationships.

Embracing the self-healing journey

Engaging in self-healing using a meaning-based story approach may lead to periods of turmoil and discomfort, including the specific challenges mentioned above. At one end of the spectrum of possibilities, you might uncover feelings that, when expressed appropriately and assertively, can resolve quickly alongside your symptoms. At the opposite extreme, you may confront deeply rooted issues that could significantly impact certain relationships. Allowing for discomfort at any part of the spectrum is important because this discomfort is not only essential for your healing, but also for your personal growth in general.

Recognizing that you hold personal responsibility for your discomfort and any associated feelings allows you to approach various situations with greater wisdom and insight. If you encounter feelings that are overwhelming or insurmountable, it's important to remain open to seeking help from a skilled therapist who can guide you through these challenges.

As we navigate the complexities of our emotional landscape, it is useful to acknowledge that the difficulties we experience with certain feelings often stem from past experiences of personal hurt or loss. These feelings are often contained in memories that cast shadows on our present, leading us to view them through a lens of fear or apprehension. Acknowledging this connection allows us to understand that while our feelings may be overwhelming now, they are rooted in our history rather than our current reality.

If there is an ageless wisdom we can turn to at this point, it is that as we are hurt in relationship, so too are we healed in relationship. This profound truth reflects the interconnectedness of all experience. Personal growth, while often fraught with difficulties, brings with it immense rewards—new insights, deeper connections, and a more authentic sense of self. Ultimately, embracing both the challenges and the benefits of this journey can lead to profound transformation and fulfillment.

Easy or difficult, it's the journey itself that matters

There is no set pace to your self-healing journey. Some people will want to move quickly, others prefer a meandering pace. Sometimes the seriousness of someone's GERD reflects the complexity of their story. But this is not always the case. There is no real way to predict how quickly or slowly we can process our personal, subjective material. How fast one moves through anything is of no importance. You will be best served to embark on your self-help journey at your own pace. As Spanish poet Antonio Machado once wrote, "Traveler, there is no path, the path is made by walking." My role simply is to remind you to keep taking steps, the exact nature of which will be unique for everyone.

You may find that you easily make connections between your story and symptoms, and may notice immediate improvements in your GERD symptoms. Having made these connections, you may not need all the assistance on offer. Or you may find that healing occurs more gradually, with symptoms improving over weeks or even months. It could be that your physical symptoms disappear, yet you feel that there is more of your story to unpack in order to resolve all the issues behind your illness.

Whatever velocity you move through life, it's only the journey itself that matters. Your unique circumstances such as your motivation and energy levels, the degree to which you identify with—or are attached to—your GERD, and the time you have had GERD will not count against you; they simply inform your journey. Anyone who is committed to holding a broad view of their illness will eventually come to see the connections between their story and symptoms.

The key message here is that rather than finding reasons as to why your symptoms might persist, you need to embrace your symptoms for the wisdom they represent. After all, your symptoms have brought you this far. The destination you are pursuing—the point at which you are healed from GERD—is unknown. The only thing that matters then is the journey, not the destination.

Exercise 3.1: Check-in for increased self-awareness

Self check-ins can be performed for a variety of reasons, including for increased self-awareness, emotional regulation, goal alignment, and encouraging self-compassion. I've included a self check-in exercise here because it's a good time to find out how you feel about this fresh perspective and whether your own GERD symptoms are flaring in response to any early connections being made with your story.

So take a moment to check in with yourself right now.

1. Start in a comfortable position, sitting or lying, in a quiet space where you won't be disturbed. Allow your body to relax, and close your eyes if you feel comfortable doing so.

2. Take a deep breath in through your nose, allowing your abdomen to expand. Hold for a moment, then exhale slowly through your mouth. Repeat this deep breathing for

three full rounds, feeling the tension in your body begin to dissipate.

3. Shift your awareness to your body, starting at the top of your head and slowly moving downwards. Notice any areas of tension or discomfort, particularly around your chest and abdomen, which may relate to your GERD. Acknowledge these sensations without judgment, just observing what you feel.

4. Now, bring your awareness to any strong feelings around your GERD. Allow these to surface without trying to change them. Simply acknowledge their presence.

5. Shift your awareness to your thoughts. What thoughts arise when you think about your GERD and a possible connection between your story and your symptoms? Observe these thoughts, recognizing them for what they are but not allowing yourself to engage with them or get swept away by them.

6. Consider what fresh insights might be available to you right now. How do these affect your understanding of your symptoms? Take a moment to reflect on how this new perspective influences your feelings about GERD and your approach moving forward.

7. In closing, take a few deep breaths, expressing gratitude toward yourself for taking this opportunity to reflect and check in. When you're ready, open your eyes and return to your surroundings.

This exercise can be revisited whenever you need to reconnect with yourself or to connect more deeply with your experiences with GERD. An alternative to this exercise is after you get to Step 5 and before you move to Step 6, ask yourself which of your significant interpersonal relationships come to mind while thinking about your symptoms? If you feel the start of panic or you need to resist what you are thinking and feeling, that is okay. Remind yourself that you are safe, that it is normal and acceptable to experience strong feelings and know that these feelings will pass.

---

1. Broom, B., (2007). Meaning-full disease: How personal experience and meanings cause and maintain physical illness. Oxfordshire, UK; Routledge.

2. Broom, B., (2013). In B. Broom (Ed.), Transforming clinical practice using the MindBody approach: A radical integration. Oxfordshire, UK; Routledge.

3. Brené Brown. The power of vulnerability. Available at: https://www.ted.com/talks/brene_brown_the_power_of_vulnerability?subtitle=en

4. Brené Brown. Listening to shame. Available at: https://www.ted.com/talks/brene_brown_listening_to_shame?subtitle=en

Four

Exploring a Meaning-Based Story Approach

Modern medicine, while excellent for treating acute illnesses and physical trauma, is ineffective at treating chronic illnesses such as GERD because it separates physical symptoms from personal experience and meaning.[1] In order to appreciate this profound limitation and to understand how a meaning-based story approach can provide a need fulfillment for you and your GERD, let's take a look at a case example. Although this example is of a person with cancer, I've chosen it for its simple elegance and impact.

James' story[2]

James (not his real name) has given me permission to share his story.

James, a 38-year-old retail manager, saw me at his wife's insistence for help dealing with the stress of his ongoing battle with testicular cancer. His chief complaint was fatigue, which began when chemotherapy was started following the removal of his diseased testis.

James was concerned that his fatigue would prevent him from completing the full course of chemotherapy. At the time of his diagnosis, James was undergoing a work redundancy, which coincided with the birth of his son. I learned that

James' son was conceived using assisted reproductive technology as a consequence of James having male factor infertility.

Telling me his story, James offered up a general feeling of battle weariness. He said, "This cancer diagnosis came as *a fair whack*," and "this cancer has been *my life*." He also told me, "I'm dreading the outcome."

When I reflected to James that his fatigue was unsurprising given his story of being in a battle for his life, James became distressed. After offering him my empathetic response to let him know that his distress was completely appropriate and good to express, we did some further healing work together.

We specifically focused on his statement of dread and explored the accompanying feelings in his body. With this shift toward his feelings, he became more noticeably relaxed.

James began our session visibly lethargic, overwhelmed with worry and believing he would never be able to complete his chemotherapy due to the fatigue he felt. But in less than an hour together, he had changed his belief and was now convinced that his remaining treatment would be a doddle. This new belief was reflected in his posture and energy levels. His face had lost some of its puffiness, and he had a breezy smile for the first time.

Medicine sees only part of James

Medicine limits doctors in how they are permitted to *see* James. Starting with what medicine does see, James' testicular cancer is explained as a harmful deviation of the testis from physicochemical norms, which produces a tumor. In other words, the tumor results from an unexplained molecular defect, which may have a genetic component but is typically understood in terms of unknown environmental factors.

Any reported symptoms, such as pain and swelling of the testis and local lymph nodes, are backed up by the doctor's physical examination. This includes palpation of the testis, the doctor's own observation (sign) of an abnormal enlargement of the affected organ, and ultrasound evaluation. Treatment involves removal of the diseased testis, which is then subjected to laboratory tests to confirm the malignancy. Chemotherapy follows to limit the spread of any remaining tumor cells.

To arrive at this diagnosis, the doctor is required to exclude James' subjective story, including that: James was diagnosed with male factor infertility two years before his cancer diagnosis; he was undergoing a workplace redundancy at the time he began to feel pain in his testis; James had been an expectant dad when his symptoms began and welcomed his newborn son into the world around the time of his cancer diagnosis; and his son was conceived using assisted reproductive technology.

These life events are all part of James' story and, most importantly, they are also part of his suffering. Yet, medicine dismisses these events as having no relationship to disease causation, diagnosis and treatment.

Three key limitations of the biomedical model

1). Medicine focuses on symptoms, not the wholeperson

Doctors are trained to have a narrow view of illness in order to work within the paradigm known as the biomedical model. This model *assumes* that the body possesses mechanical properties, which, when considered as a whole, resembles a machine. The body-machine can be reduced to a series of parts, knowledge of which is used to understand individual signs and symptoms that arise when one or more of the parts breaks down. Like any machine, the body is considered to be prone to such breakdowns, particularly as it ages. And like a mechanic, the doctor is not concerned with other "healthy parts" except to exclude them from having any role in causing our symptoms.

Signs and symptoms are believed to result from a physical abnormality within the body compartment, which is considered to be separate from the mind compartment and a person's subjective experiences. If this physical abnormality affects brain chemistry, this is used to explain mental suffering and illness. If this physical abnormality affects any other part of the body, this is used to explain physical illness.

Relating these assumptions to James' circumstances, biomedicine regards his signs and symptoms as a deviation of his body's normal function. James' doctors are trained to look at his testicular cancer as being separate from James the person. We can say that biomedicine sees James' testicular cancer as a disease-object which arises through the mechanical dysfunction of the body-object. The symptoms of the body-object become the doctor's sole focus and James, the wholeperson, is excluded from the clinical encounter.[3]

2). Medicine separates mind from body

The biomedical model emerged during the industrial revolution from a now 400-year-old assumption that mind is somehow separate from the body. Since then, biomedicine has adopted a slightly different assumption, which holds that the mind is a secondary product of the body and is located to a specific part of the brain. In this way, biomedicine has retained its dualistic origins by suggesting that our subjective experience arises only because, as humans, we have a highly developed brain which produces consciousness, with the body having primacy (first cause).

"Physical" things are considered to be separate from the mind. In the biomedical model, these physical things are thought of as real and therefore permitted. In contrast, a person's subjective story and any associated feelings are not permitted since they are a product of our individual consciousness and therefore distinct or separate from the body.

Again, relating these assumptions to James, the biomedical model ignores his past experience of male factor infertility, and current workplace redundancy and expectant fatherhood status because there are no causally related physical symptoms. Although his infertility involved the same organ part as his cancer, there is no direct causal evidence to connect these two events other than through unknown genetic, developmental or environmental factors.

3). Medicine dismisses the personal narrative that always accompanies chronic illness

In James' case, his mental suffering and emotional anguish must have been immense to endure two years of constant setbacks that challenged the core of his masculinity. Yet this aspect of his suffering is excluded from having any causative or even contributory role to his testicular cancer because any illness must always be explained in its physical terms. This despite the possible meaning for James' disease staring his doctors in the face!

The bottom line is that in medicine today, you and I—wholepersons—are regarded as having no participatory role in either causing or overcoming our illness. Only the body-machine in concert with drugs, surgery, other medical interventions, and possibly diet and exercise can manifest any sort of healing. In contrast, spontaneous healing when it occurs is regarded as the exception to the rule, and is not permitted to be explained in any way other than chance.

Effects of the medical model on treatment outcomes

These profound limitations of medicine are best summarized in philosophical terms. Our current medical model[4] requires doctors to consider mind and body as separate parts or compartments. As such, there can be no meaningful interactions between them: Thoughts cannot create things; matter is always above mind; there is no room for personal subjectivity or the unique story that evolves from an individual's conscious experiences. There is no room for personal meaning.

Too many doctors today regrettably persist with the idea that mechanistic medicine is the only kind that works.[5] Unfortunately, many alternative practitioners succumb to the same conditioning that has produced the biomedical model, offering alternative physical treatments that similarly fail to acknowledge a person's underlying subjectivity and which may be no better, and potentially even less effective, than conventional medicine.

The most obvious outcome of this restricted thinking is in the way new industries continue to blossom from our need for symptomatic relief. Vast industries in the fields of aging, cosmetics, exercise physiology, genetics, nutraceuticals, nutrition and others have joined with the pharmaceutical industry in aiming to perfect new products intended to ease our physical discomfort. Meanwhile, as long as our subjective stories remain unaddressed, these often innovative solutions will fall short of the end to suffering that we demand from them. As long as we continue to focus solely on our symptoms, we will only ever have a superficial experience of life, and more symptoms.

The MindBody solution

"A fair whack"

At the precise moment that James said, "a fair whack," I closed my legs in empathy as one man does for another when the first describes a painful blow to his testes [ouch@!]. It is not my intention to be crude. It is true, if you will pardon the pun, that James' story throws a great punch. But my main intention is to use his case to show how meaning, when observed, is important not only to the individual whose story *carries* the meaning. It is also important to a receptive listener who is open to the meaning in another person's story.

Indeed, when an active listener grasps the possible hidden meaning in another person's words, and responds in an empathetic way, this will often help the storyteller to recognize the deeper meaning in their own story. Two things helped me to make an immediate connection between James' exact words and his cancer: First, I was listening actively for *somatic metaphor*; and second, I was using my own body as a sounding board for the resonance of James' words.

Somatic metaphor and its embodied resonances

Somatic metaphor is a useful place to start. Literally meaning *body story*, somatic metaphor is unconsciously expressed and occurs when a person's story appears to *say* or symbolize the same thing as their physical symptoms. Thus, James' literal statement that his cancer came as "a fair whack" seemed to be symbolic of the physical disease present in his testis.

This is useful to understanding GERD: Paying attention to somatic metaphor allows us to quickly make connections between our actual words and our physical symptoms.

When you become consciously attuned to your own and others' words, the next skill is to *listen* deeply for the synchronous resonance of these words in your body. Think of your body as a tuning fork and yourself as a master musician. A master musician *knows* when the right note is struck because they feel the resonance of that note in a precise location of their body. This resonant aspect of our story is important because, as self-healers, it helps us to bring any meaning that is unconsciously held in the bodymind into its full conscious expression. This facilitates emotional, psychological *and* physical transformation.

This resonance also helps the listener, such as a therapist, to attune to the root of another person's distress. It is a simple enough practice and anyone who gets better at attuning to their own body can acquire the useful skill of *listening* for the embodied resonances of other people's stories. I believe this skill is critical to teach and to learn if all therapeutic relationships are to be healing relationships. This overlooked capacity of one human to connect with another through the whole of our being enables the sufferer to feel seen, heard and held, bringing them back to connection.

"This cancer has been my life"

Coming back to James' story, he also said, "This cancer has been my life." At face value, James' words might convey the meaning that his recent life was filled with cancer concerns from diagnosis, hospital and clinic visits, anticancer treatments and their side effects, and worrying about his own and his family's future.

But I intuited that James' words held a much deeper meaning. I felt that he was communicating unconsciously—through his exact words—a deeper story involving a much longer struggle. And given the nature of the cancer in his testis, I felt that the struggle he was trying to communicate involved his masculine identity. Taking this idea further, I believed that he had unconsciously embodied his masculine identity in his testes, which had taken on the form—and come to symbolize—his life's struggles.

At this point in our conversation, I began to hold James' testicular cancer as a possible symbolic representation of three key ideas overlooked by the biomedical model. Specifically, these were of James' story of male factor infertility, workplace redundancy, and expectant fatherhood of a child he had conceived with his wife only through the intervention of assisted reproductive technology.

Gently testing the waters, I asked James if he would like to explore these aspects of his story in relation to his cancer. James declined the invitation, preferring to focus on his elevated energy levels now he no longer felt the fatigue that only moments before had threatened to derail his treatment.

Exploring the psychosocial origins of James' cancer

I later reflected on Western gender stereotypes and particularly on society's expectations of men as being virile and potent providers whose chief role is to project confidence and power while bringing status, strength and abundance to their families. I know from my own experiences of masculinity that this messaging is incredibly damaging to young boys and men.

Today, I believe that a person's illness is an unconscious response that is explained, at least in part, by the destructive limitations that society imposes on its citizens through unhelpful messaging, especially in the media and classrooms. My view is that James' mind-story and body-symptoms are an unconscious rebellion against a masculine gender role that emphasizes a certain type of manhood at the expense of a more balanced masculinity. The tension between James' self-identity and family and societal expectations around the ideal male produced an inner conflict out of which his testicular cancer emerged as a messenger urging conscious action.

With society's continuing emphasis on unattainable ideals that resonate just as much for women as men,[6] James is unlikely to be alone in his unconscious rebellion. Again, using the example of James' testicular cancer, his experience is not an isolated one. Studies investigating issues of masculinity among men living with cancer unsurprisingly focused on prostate and testicular cancers. The title of one of these research reports was, "It's hard to take because I am a man's man."[7] The title of another was, "It's caveman stuff, but that is to a certain extent how guys still operate."[8] Similar ethnographic studies have been published for women living with breast cancer and speak to the emotional, social and relational aspects of the disease, as well as personal identity. One of these was titled, "I had to make them feel at ease."[9] The title of another: "I've been through something."[10]

Meaningful yes, meanings' fundamentalism no

Again, using James' case as a specific example, a word of caution is appropriate. The Western ethnographic view of testicular cancer may not be appropriate for other cultures, nor indeed for all men with this cancer in Western society. It may be inappropriate to hold a Western cultural perspective if a person with testicular cancer was, for example, East Asian and practiced Taoism as a religion. A man with a Taoist perspective is unlikely to view his testicular cancer in terms of the yang (masculine) qualities seen in Western perspectives. Rather, he would likely view the testis in terms of its yin (feminine) qualities. These qualities include patience, supportiveness, solidity, reliability and resourcefulness typical of an organ used for production, storage, and conservation. Other cultures will have their own unique cultural biases that can give rise to other ethnographic descriptors and even somatic metaphors.

Although James' story appeared to be meaningful from my perspective, it is important to remember that in considering someone else's story, it is their own subjective interpretation that determines meaning. Because every individual living with disease will have a different story, we cannot always expect to find the same meaning even if the disease is the same.

However, I believe that we can always use a person's story to explain the cause of disease. As a consequence, our story and physical symptoms no longer need to compete for our attention. This comes with the caveat that understanding our disease in a meaningful way is possible only when we allow the story in the same *space* as we allow our symptoms.

A meaningful outcome

Following the removal of his diseased testis, and the completion of chemotherapy which resulted in remission of the cancer, James became a stay-at-home dad. He embraced the opportunity to raise his infant son while his wife became the breadwinner. James resolved the inner conflict that his disease had flagged to him by reconciling his own masculinity with the noble and mature masculine qualities of supportiveness, solidity, reliability and resourcefulness.

Exercise 4.1: Shifting awareness to subjective suffering

Let's use this meaning-based story approach while shifting perspective back toward your GERD and its subjective aspect in particular. This exercise is really about having a conversation with yourself to uncover the feelings and thoughts you have about your GERD, which in turn might point to its meaning for you. One of the ways you can do this is to reflect on each of the symptoms of GERD that are most bothersome, then write down or record any insights that you have. But instead of focusing exclusively on the physical sensations of your symptoms, this exercise requires you to broaden your perspective to include the subjective aspects of your suffering.

For example, if I asked you what is it like to experience heartburn after eating your favorite meal, you might initially think of the feeling or sensation of the heartburn before beginning to relate to me the subjective qualities of: Why your favorite meal is your favorite meal; how it effects you not being able to truly enjoy your favorite meal knowing that it won't be long until you experience heartburn; how your feeling of heartburn might be the same or different to someone else's experience; and what it would mean to you if you didn't have to worry about heartburn anymore.

The exercise works best when you follow your intuition, avoid censoring any responses you think of, and be prepared to cast your net wide. Here are some examples of other questions that you might ask yourself:

What is it like to...

- Taste the acid of your stomach in your mouth?

- Experience the pain of GERD in your chest or abdomen?

- Avoid your favorite foods for fear of the consequences?

- Worry that someone will be offended by your belching or bad breath?

- Wake up in the middle of the night with a cough that won't go away?

- Wake up in the morning, every morning, without having had a refreshing night's rest?

- Speak in a croaky voice or have the feeling of something catching in your throat?

If you struggle to relate to this exercise, return to the example of James and put yourself in his shoes. How else might he describe the experience of cancer if he was pressed to relate it to a whole-of-life struggle rather than the narrow window of time since he had symptoms? If cancer really had been his life as he suggested, what might it have been like growing up as a male in his family? You might come up with terms such as invalidating, performance-focused and defensiveness, as well as feelings such as inadequacy, insecurity, isolation and anger.

Now, extending the same level of empathy toward your situation that you would use to understand someone else's perspective, take a moment to reflect on your own struggle. What words and feelings can you use to describe it? Write down or in some other way record your thoughts and feelings.

Exercise 4.2: Journaling as you journey

Writing down or in some other way recording your thoughts, feelings and experiences is immeasurably useful for anyone on a personal growth journey. For someone with GERD or another illness, journaling is a powerful therapeutic tool. By diligently keeping a journal or workbook, before long you will have a number of thoughts, memories and feelings that you can return to at any time. Here's a step-by-step guide to help you get started:

1. **Choosing your journal:** Select a journal that resonates with you. This could be a traditional notebook, a document on your computer, a digital app, a voice recorder, or creating a visual record using a camera. Make sure whatever format you select feels right for you.

2. **Setting a regular time for journaling:** Decide on a time that fits into your daily routine. Consistency helps make journaling a positive habit.

3. **Creating a welcoming space:** Find a quiet, comfortable place to journal, such as a cozy corner of your home or a peaceful spot outdoors. Make sure the space you choose for your journaling is free of unwelcome distractions.

4. **Starting with a prompt:** Begin your journaling sessions with a specific prompt. This could be the same prompt each time, such as "What did I eat today, and how did I feel afterwards?" Or it could be a unique prompt based on a specific experience you've had since your last journaling session. As well as asking yourself "What?" questions such as "What feelings do I experience when I have GERD symptoms?" remember to ask yourself the harder "Why?" questions too: "Why do I feel blah after eating chocolate?" or "Why do I

feel anxious around dinner time?"

5. **Reflecting on your experiences:** After journaling your latest experiences, take a moment to reflect. How do these experiences connect? Are there any patterns you notice in your symptoms, the foods you've eaten, your emotional responses? For example: "I noticed that I feel more anxious when I eat out, and my symptoms are often worse than usual afterwards. I wonder why that is? Things are a bit tight financially, but it feels good to reward myself with a night off cooking once in a while."

6. **Tracking your symptoms:** Incorporate a habit of journaling your GERD symptoms. For example: "Symptoms: Mild heartburn after breakfast, stressed about work." In a later chapter, *Charting your symptoms*, I include an example chart used to track your symptoms and mood shifts over time.

7. **Writing freely:** Allow yourself the freedom to journal about anything that comes to mind. Journaling is a personal space, so express your thoughts freely, including those that are seemingly unrelated to your GERD. For example: "I'm grateful for the support of my friends, even when I can't join them for dinner."

8. **Reviewing and reflecting regularly:** Schedule regular times—weekly or monthly—to review your past entries. Look for patterns, themes and other possible insights. This often aids in meaning-making.

Remember, journaling is a journey. As you build a collection of entries, you may begin to have insights around personal meaning that was previously hidden. This process of meaning-making can empower you to explore the different layers of story through which deeper healing is accessed. Celebrate your progress, no matter how small, and trust that regular journaling will deepen your understanding and provide clarity over time. Keep going—you're taking a significant step toward self-awareness and healing your GERD!

---

1. Broom, B., (2007). Meaning-*full* disease: How personal experience and meanings cause and maintain physical illness. Oxfordshire, UK; Routledge.

2. Christian, H.B., (2015). Subjective dimensions of meaning in the clinical encounter: Unifying personhood and disease. *Energy Psychology: Theory, Research and Treatment*, 7(1): 30–38.

3. Shalom, A., (1989). The body/mind conceptual framework and the problem of personal identity: Some theories in philosophy, psychoanalysis & neurology. Atlantic Highlands, NJ, USA; Humanities Press International, Inc.

4. The biopsychosocial (BPS) model, developed in the 1970s as an alternative to the biomedical model, attempts to address some of the limitations of the latter. The BPS model expands upon the biomedical perspective by incorporating psychological, social, and environmental factors as influences on the body-machine. However, in practice, the BPS model changes little; doctors are still restricted to interpreting a patient's illness solely in physical terms, without taking into account the patient's personal narrative.

5. Sheldrake, R., (2012). The science delusion: Freeing the spirit of enquiry. London, UK; Coronet.

6. I'm thinking of the impossible standards placed on women in society to balance the various ideals of womanhood as: Nurturer and caregiver; homemaker and professional achiever; glamor icon and visual siren; emotional caretaker and social connector; and mindful parent and disciplined educator.

7. Cecil, R., McCaughan, E., & Parahoo, K., (2010). "It's hard to take because I am a man's man": An ethnographic exploration of cancer and masculinity. *European Journal of Cancer*, 19(4): 501-509.

8. O'Brien, R., Hunt, K., & Hart, G., (2005). "It's caveman stuff, but that is to a certain extent how guys still operate": Men's accounts of masculinity and help seeking. *Social Science and Medicine*, 61(3): 503-516.

9. Wright, J. D., Kroenke, C. H., Kwan, M. L., Kushi, L. H., (2021). "I had to make them feel at ease": Narrative accounts of how women with breast cancer navigate social support. *Qualitative Health Research*, 31(6): 1056-1068.

10. Kooken, W. C., Haase, J. E., & Russell, K. M., (2007). "I've been through something": Poetic explorations of African American women's cancer survivorship. *Western Journal of Nursing Research*, 29(7): 896-919.

Five

Skepticism is Welcome: Addressing Your Hesitancy

Objections to a meaning-based story approach

Having doubts at the moment? I can relate! Back in 2006, when I was first exposed to the MindBody paradigm as Dr. Brian Broom's patient,[1,2,3] I felt a little put out. Brian asked me what else was going on in my life when I first experienced hay fever symptoms. He knew I was an immunologist, having met previously at a conference, yet here he was asking me to set aside my detailed understanding of allergies to discuss something deeply personal that I thought had nothing to do with my lifelong struggle with hay fever. A quick glance outside his window that fine spring morning revealed all the evidence I needed to justify my symptoms; nature's verdant bounty in full bloom. Pollen was my sworn enemy—along with dust mites, animal dander, mould spores, insect stings, dairy...

Fortunately, Brian had faced sterner tests in his career as a consultant immunologist and psychotherapist. He'd learned over years of clinical practice how to engage the skeptics, cynics and the weary. More importantly, he knew how to disarm his medical colleagues and allied health scientists enough to secure their referrals. In my life experiences and role within the pharmaceutical industry, I had crossed into all these territories.

When first introduced to the idea that a person's illness relates to their subjective story, it's natural to have questions. A strong reaction to this may stem from dogma, as it did for me, but can also arise from a misunderstanding.

Perhaps you had a negative experience with the medical profession when you were told your symptoms were psychosomatic or "all in your head." The use of this unfortunate label is not uncommon and ties back to how doctors are trained to perceive symptoms.

Some people quickly accept that their story plays a role in their GERD but worry about the implications. Because story is viewed as a mental construct, fears may arise that symptoms are purely psychological or that someone is to blame for their illness. Others, like me, find it hard to accept that their story impacts physical health, preferring "more scientific," data-driven explanations for their illnesses.[4]

In my brief sessions with Brian, brought on by my second attempt at allergy desensitization—which, like my first as a child, would ultimately fail—I realized that the limited evidence for MindBody practice was not as significant a problem as the restrictive philosophy of conventional medicine. Through Brian, I learned a great deal about philosophy, but my early reluctance to embrace a meaning-based story approach delayed my healing. I guess I had to navigate life the hard way.

Today, when someone asks me, "Where is your evidence?" I respond, "Philosophy offers a deeper truth that no amount of data can touch."

GERD is not "all in your head"

When considering the role of your story in physical disease, this does not mean that your symptoms are all in your head, nor do they indicate that you are a hypochondriac or mentally weak. Most people can agree that everyone experiences stress in some form within their body. This is not a contentious statement because we have all felt the rapid heartbeat that accompanies conflict or threats to our safety. In moments of heightened awareness, you may notice physical responses—such as a dry mouth, prickling skin as the tiny hairs on your body stand up, or sweaty palms.

Consider this: If I told you a story about a man who accidentally killed his young child in a driveway vehicle accident and who subsequently developed cancer in the months afterward, you would likely agree that stress played a role in his disease. Where you might draw the line, however, is accepting that his overwhelming grief and guilt contributed to his disease.

The reality is that we all experience stress differently. Some people experience stress as *gut* disturbances, others may get headaches or skin complaints, while some may develop high blood pressure. Stress is a universal phenomenon, and without our bodies we would not even recognize it. Even those who claim to be in perfect health carry stress and its narrative within them.

> You are reading this book because you or someone you care about has GERD. Your symptoms are real—they manifest in your body. No one can claim that your symptoms are imaginary.

The challenge arises in recognizing that our experience of a physical illness like GERD is unique to everyone with the disease. In addition to the observable signs and symptoms, we experience a subjective quality that reflects the unique aspects of our suffering. There is no easy way of measuring this aspect of GERD. Yet it is *always* a part of our disease.

If you consider yourself stable and free from major life traumas, you may think that your story is irrelevant to your GERD. However, I encourage you to look beyond any resistance you might feel. Admitting to personal issues that are expressed through your body requires a significant degree of vulnerability, which can feel intimidating, particularly for men.

Now, contemplate this question: Is it more valuable to have GERD that a doctor can see and treat, yet not resolve? Or is it better to have GERD caused by underlying emotional issues that affect your well-being and quality of life as long as you remain unwilling to explore your story?

Accepting your vulnerability and leaping into the unknown takes courage. The reward for this leap is personal growth and expanded opportunities for an enriched and abundant life.

Understanding disease does not require blame

Some people worry that connecting their personal story to their GERD symptoms implies that someone else, like a parent, must take the blame. This common concern arises from a simplistic perspective of illness. However, just as we compassionately recognize the unintended consequences faced by the man who accidentally ran over his child, we must extend the same compassion to ourselves and the other people who accompany us on our life's journey.

We never consciously intend to harm others, nor can we reliably predict how our actions might affect someone else's well-being, or vice versa. If you find yourself grappling with feelings of blame related to your GERD, remember that disease—as for any form of suffering—arises from multiple contributing factors. No single cause or person is solely to blame.

> Rather than apportioning blame, we can view our disease as an opportunity to heal troubled relationships, including the one we have with ourselves.

Disease is not just about genetics

While our genes do play a role in the development of GERD and related disorders,[5] the narrative that has evolved over recent decades often places undue emphasis on genetic factors. Media coverage frequently highlights genetics as the culprit for various conditions, including GERD, as diseases like personality traits tend to run in families.

But it is a misconception to believe that our genes dictate our fate. Genes are not the ultimate rulers of our lives that we once believed them to be; rather, they are responsive to environmental cues for their activation and deactivation. Although genetics are important in determining our susceptibility to GERD, they alone do not cause the disease.

Therefore, we would benefit more from examining the environmental triggers that play a significant role in our GERD.[6] A meaning-based story approach to your GERD acknowledges the subjective dimensions of personal meaning as environmental triggers, giving you the opportunity to take over as governor of your life.[7]

A common scenario in medicine

If you remain skeptical of arguments that challenge the assumptions underlying modern medicine, consider this scenario:

Imagine that I am as comfortable today as I was in 2006 with the idea that a person's illness can be explained solely by its physical signs and symptoms. It's important to distinguish between these two terms: Signs are objectively observed—measured by someone other than the patient—whereas symptoms are subjective, relying on the patient's self-report.

Now suppose that four weeks ago I was involved in an incident during which a mugger held a knife to my throat. In the intervening time, I've had some help from a crisis counselor, but have noticed some persistent physical discomfort that hasn't come up in our counseling sessions. So I decide to see my doctor.

Having my doctor accept my symptom report at face value is key to obtaining a diagnosis. A diagnosis is therefore a negotiation, but only in the sense that my symptoms are helpful cues that direct the doctor toward the relevant signs that are needed for them to make an accurate diagnosis.

For instance, if I report symptoms like headache, tiredness, and blurred vision, my doctor may suspect high blood pressure, with its signs confirmed through a physical examination using a blood pressure cuff. If follow-up tests show persistent elevation, my doctor may diagnose hypertension.

However, if the examination reveals no physical signs to support my symptom report, the doctor might attribute my discomfort to stress. In that case, I may feel that my suffering has been unjustly dismissed. What then? We might have a short conversation about stress. Ironically, this conversation would likely yield valuable subjective insights, including the source of my current stress and my coping strategies.

Conversely, when both my doctor and I agree on my symptoms—because the corresponding signs of illness are present—I feel validated. I might receive prescribed blood pressure medication, but aside from taking the pills and a couple of counseling sessions, I have done nothing to address the subjective aspect of my distress that led me to seek medical help in the first place!

Consciousness phenomena unexplained by medicine

Many objective, measurable phenomena of consciousness remain unexplained within our mainstream worldview. Consider the following examples:

- **Near-Death Experiences (NDEs):** Nine percent of cardiac arrest survivors report having a near-death experience, with two percent providing explicit details about their NDE—despite being unconscious—related to events surrounding their resuscitation.[8]

- **Heart transplant recipients**: Heart transplant recipients often report developing new personality traits that subsequent investigations reveal belonged to their donors.[9] Anecdotal evidence includes recipients unexpectedly acquiring artistic talents or changing their dietary and gender preferences.

- **Placebo and nocebo effects**: Medicine struggles to explain the placebo effect, in which a treatment without therapeutic value produces health benefits due to the patient's belief in its efficacy. Conversely, the nocebo effect occurs when a person experiences negative health outcomes from a treatment that poses no real harm, driven by the belief that it is harmful.[10]

In addition to these phenomena, medicine fails to account for numerous other aspects of consciousness, often dismissing them as side notes. Yet, their existence—whether individually or collectively—compels us to reconsider our understanding of reality and our true nature. Here are just a few more examples of consciousness phenomena that merit serious consideration:

- Mind and body interactions.

- Emotional influences on physical health.

- Spontaneous remission.

- Subjective conscious experiences based on our sensory perceptions.

- The health benefits of volunteering, including increased longevity.

- Adverse childhood experiences (ACEs), which can lead to physical and mental diseases in adults, independent of lifestyle factors.

- The effectiveness of healing practices from various traditions, such as Traditional Chinese Medicine and acupuncture.

- The common experience of synchronicity, where seemingly unrelated events appear to be causally connected.

The whole of you

When we consider the connection between our stories and symptoms, we open the door to healing mind, body, and soul. This perspective allows us to explore causes of disease beyond just genetic molecular aberrations and unknown developmental and environmental factors. Specifically, it helps us integrate meaning with our illness, potentially resolving unconscious conflicts and leading us to a sense of wholeness.[11]

This approach is variously termed a MindBody, integrated or wholeperson perspective, and which I have termed a meaning-based story approach. It embodies a unified understanding of the body and mind, where both matter (body) and energy (mind) co-emerge from a foundation of consciousness.[12] Within this framework, attempting to separate the body and mind becomes meaningless due to their deep entanglement. The wholeperson perspective also brings together the different facets of "I," preventing their separation, categorization, or compartmentalization.

For instance, saying "I am physical" captures one aspect of the whole, but it does not negate other aspects that coexist within the same space. Thus, statements like "I am conscious," "I am emotional," "I am feeling," "I am thoughtful," "I am relational," "I am soulful," and "I am spiritual" are all equally valid expressions of the overarching "I Am," without needing separate compartments for each.

This seamless understanding of the wholeperson embraces a unity of being that resonates with human experience and holds intuitive strength. The meaning-based story approach reflects all the ways we describe ourselves without giving precedence to any single aspect. It retains familiar descriptors of human experience while encouraging us to view one aspect (e.g., our thoughts) as integrally connected to another (e.g., our body).

With its emphasis on *being*, the meaning-based story approach allows for a comprehensive understanding. We can carve the whole into its parts when needed to describe different facets of our being. But a deeper unity prevails in which the "I Am" is irreducible. We are always at once physical, mental, and subjective (conscious) in our being.

A unitary reality

Accepting this unitary reality of the wholeperson brings consequences.

First, we are not a passive passenger in life whose biology in concert with a hostile environment determines our reality. Rather, we construct our own reality through interactions involving our different "I Am" facets in concert with a self-reflective environment.

Second, the language we use to describe our reality is enriched by our sense of "I Am-ness," and is inseparable from the whole. Our words then are deeply embodied, and we engage our entire being when we speak—it's as if words "speak us" more so than we speak words.

Third, disease arises from this "I Am-ness," allowing us to perceive its physical and subjective dimensions. Meaning also emerges from broader contexts, including familial, relational, sociocultural, environmental, and spiritual aspects.

The diseased or disturbed "I Am" reflects specific patterns in our lives, understood only by exploring these patterns from multiple perspectives. Meaning unfolds when we overlay the physical and subjective experiences of life. Relating the disturbed "I Am" back to story offers various entry points:

- **Story in language**: For example, expressing anger through words.

- **Story in writing and literature**: Recording private thoughts and feelings in a diary.

- **Story in non-verbal communication**: Conveying defensiveness through posture.

- **Story in action**: Working out grief through activities like running.

- **Story in art, drama, and music**: Using mediums such as painting or mime to express feelings of disgust or abandonment.

- **Story in the body**: How James' disturbed "I Am" manifested, and how your own "I Am" appears in your GERD.

When you are ready to embrace the multidimensional nature of your being, you can start the process of restoring the disturbed "I Am" to wholeness. "I Am" evolves into "I Am One."

In achieving this, your experience with suffering and disease no longer diminishes you. Instead, through meaning, you find value, strength, and purpose. As you grow through this journey, your ability to connect with others in new and meaningful ways also expands. Your awareness of self, family and community is enhanced. "I Am One" becomes "We Are One."

I hope this section of the book has allayed any concerns you have about how story relates to your GERD while sparking your own perspectives on why we can all benefit from a new understanding of disease. In the next section, we'll explore personal meaning more closely to better understand the relationship between GERD and your story.

1. Broom, B., (1997). Somatic illness and the patient's other story. London, UK; Free Association Books.

2. Broom, B., (2007). Meaning-*full* disease: How personal experience and meanings cause and maintain physical illness. Oxfordshire, UK; Routledge.

3. Broom, B., (2013). In B. Broom (Ed.), Transforming clinical practice using the MindBody approach: A radical integration. Oxfordshire, UK; Routledge.

4. Beauregard, M., Schwartz, G.E., Miller, L., Dossey, L., Moreira-Almeida, A., Schlitz, M., Sheldrake, R., & Tart, C., (2014). Manifesto for a post-materialist science. Available at: https://opensciences.org/files/pdfs/Manifesto-for-a-Post-Materialist-Science.pdf

5. Argyrou, A., Legaki, E., Koutserimpas, C., Gazouli, M., Papaconstantinou, I., Gkiokas, G., & Karamanolis, G., (2018). Risk factors for gastroesophageal reflux disease and analysis of genetic contributors. *World Journal of Clinical Cases,* 6(8): 176-182.

6. Church, D., (2007). The genie in your genes: Epigenetic medicine and the new biology of intention. Santa Rosa, CA, USA; Elite Books.

7. Christian, H.B., (2015). Subjective dimensions of meaning in the clinical encounter: Unifying personhood and disease. *Energy Psychology: Theory, Research and Treatment,* 7(1): 30–38.

8. Parnia, S., Spearpoint, K., de Vos, G., Fenwick, P., Goldberg, D., Yang, J., Zhu, J., Baker, K., Killingback, H., McLean, P., Wood, M., Zafari, A.M., Dickert, N., Beisteiner, R., Sterz, F., Berger, M., Warlow, C., Bullock, S., Lovett, S., Metcalfe Smith McPara, R., et al., (2014). AWARE – AWAreness during Resuscitation – a prospective study. *Resuscitation,* 85(12): 1799-1805.

9. Dossey, L., (2008). Transplants, cellular memory, and reincarnation. *Explore,* 4(5): 285-293.

10. Arnold, M. H., Finniss, D. G., & Kerridge, I., (2014). Medicine's inconvenient truth: The placebo and nocebo effect. *Internal Medicine Journal,* 44(4): 398-405.

11. Sanford, J.A., (1977). Healing and wholeness. New York, NY, USA; Paulist Press.

12. Broom, B.C., Booth, R.J., & Schubert, C., (2012). Symbolic diseases and "mindbody" co-emergence. A challenge for psychoneuroimmunology. *Explore (NY),* 8(1): 16-25.

Part II: Disease and Story

"The central question of a warrior's training is not how we avoid uncertainty and fear, but how we relate to discomfort."

— Pema Chödrön, The Places that Scare You

Six

Symptoms, Story and Meaning

Understanding meaning

Meaning emerges from our basic human need for *connection*. It comes from a deeply rooted and personal source, and not from any superficial or daily reality; rather, we have to actively look for it in order for meaning to resound in our lives.

Meaning is often described as a psychological need. It is the "ways that we make sense of ourselves and our environment, the feelings that are aroused when these understandings are constructed or violated, and the common ways in which we respond to these violations."[1] Another commentator defines meaning as "finding our purpose in our particular corner of the dark wood."[2] The existentialist philosopher Albert Camus said we find meaning in what he called "the nostalgia for unity."[3] This is the sense of once having been part of a greater whole. We experience separation from this whole as the "fundamental impulse of the human drama."

Separation from wholeness brings forth our inner dramas, while finding meaning offers the clearest path to reconnection. This is the essence of healing.

Vignette 1: A medical narrative

My own GERD started out with symptoms of heartburn, abdominal discomfort and bad breath. I began taking antacids, which gave me some relief but nothing lasting more than a couple of hours. When I developed a nighttime cough and interrupted sleep, I sought my doctor's advice.

Immediately suspecting GERD, he ordered a barium x-ray at the radiology clinic and prescribed a short course of the proton pump inhibitor, omeprazole. He also advised me to put a tilt on my bed at the head end, his suggestion for a lifestyle intervention.

The x-ray confirmed there was anatomical damage to the lower esophageal sphincter (LES) muscle. The diagnosis of GERD was confirmed when I experienced immediate relief from my symptoms after taking omeprazole.

For the next five years, I managed my disease with this once-daily tablet. If I missed a dose, the sharp symptomatic reprise reminded me to keep taking the medication as prescribed.

Vignette 2: A personal narrative

I was thirty-two when I developed GERD. My symptoms began soon after my wife became pregnant with our first child at a time when I was struggling to get some financial momentum in my new business. Our child was planned, but I felt increasingly panicked as my wife's due date and work end date drew closer. We would no longer be able to rely on her as our main breadwinner, and my business was not providing us with enough income to live on.

No sense from nonsense

After years of deeply listening to people discuss their health problems—whether family, friends, clients, or even strangers—I've noticed a common tendency to adopt the "medical narrative." This reflects how closely we align ourselves with the medical paradigm, diligently learning its terminology. We often describe our symptoms, the doctor's responses, and the processes of diagnosis and management with a significant degree of emotional detachment.

This clinical approach extends to discussions about the effects of medications, including their side effects, and the consequences of missing a dose. It seems as though we become dissociated from our bodies when we talk about our ailments.

I believe this detachment arises from the high value society—and particularly the healthcare system—places on symptoms. From a young age, we learn what interests our doctors and what does not, internalizing these values as if they are our own. These same values are continuously reinforced in various settings.

Consider my statement that "the diagnosis of GERD was confirmed when I experienced immediate relief from my symptoms after taking omeprazole." This is a clear example of the tail wagging the dog in medicine, with a pathology granted official recognition only after its symptoms respond favorably to a proposed treatment. Yet the intervention fails to address the underlying cause of the disease, a reality that becomes evident when treatment is withdrawn, leading to the return of symptoms.

Finding meaning requires endeavor and detour

In the first vignette, my doctor might have found my symptom report meaningful since his job was to make a diagnosis using objective (measurable) signs and subjective (patient-reported) symptoms. But this medically-oriented experience held no personal meaning for me:

- This meaning was manufactured from a paradigm that excludes the person from having any part in their own meaning-making, with any meaning directed at the disease rather than the person, as well as the doctor who makes the diagnosis.

- This meaning arrived without having to find purpose, make sense of myself, my feelings or my environment, or address any aspect of my basic drive for connection.

- This meaning came from a cursory evaluation of signs and symptoms, which are always a superficial representation of any underlying illness or disease.

Considered alone, our signs and symptoms can never bring us to wholeness. Story apart from bodily symptoms does not leave room for the wholeperson.

Conversely, in the second vignette where I acknowledge my personal struggles around the onset of my GERD symptoms, there is every possibility of discovering something personally meaningful from my experience. The meaning emerges naturally from the language of the storyteller, and it is our responsibility to unearth it when we know how.

This often requires endeavor and detour. The remainder of this book is therefore dedicated to uncovering the fascinating connections between your own story and GERD, then using this understanding for profound reconnection and healing.

Four sentences to direct your awareness

Returning to my personal narrative, you may find this second vignette more relatable than the previous, detached account of my symptoms. But I would like you to consider more than just relatability. If you examine each of the four sentences of my personal narrative in turn, you will notice that they give key insights using a meaning-based story approach. Specifically, they provide precise clues as to what might have caused my GERD. Remember how we briefly touched upon the idea of *somatic metaphor* or body story in the chapter, *Exploring a meaning-based story approach*? Somatic metaphor is an entry point to understanding GERD. So what message was my body trying to convey?

- "I was thirty-two when I developed GERD."

The first sentence sets the scene, providing useful demographic information that alerts the reader to life stage and what might therefore be happening in the life of a 32-year old, besides developing GERD.

- "My symptoms began soon after my wife became pregnant with our first child at a time when I was struggling to get some financial **momentum** in my new business."

This is confirmed in the second sentence, where the reader discovers that the narrator is a husband, expectant father and new business owner. We might deduce from this limited information that the narrator has a fair amount on his plate. He specifically mentions his struggle with finances, but his use of the word momentum is the most interesting detail. When we consider that he has GERD—a disease of the stomach and esophagus—the word "momentum" may or may not reference these organs in a somatic or embodied way.

The latin root of the word "momentum" comes from the verb "to move." The narrator's concern for finances parallels the idea of movement; just as financial momentum involves a state of flow, the digestive process can be seen in the same way. Once food enters the stomach, a series of processes initiate a continuous flow that enables efficient digestion and nutrient absorption. This momentum is crucial for effective digestion.

- "Our child was planned, but I felt increasingly panicked as my wife's due date and work end date drew closer."

We gain a deeper understanding of the narrator's struggle, which now connects two significant events involving his wife. We can note his fear and loss of self-agency as he looks to the future as a first-time father, and to his wife leaving her work. His potentially anxious attachment to fatherhood is understandable, but his anxiety around his wife leaving her job bears closer examination.

- "We would no longer be able to rely on her as our main **breadwinner**, and my business was not **providing** us with **enough** income to live on."

> The narrator gives very precise information here in the form of three independent metaphors that all connect his financial struggle with the stomach. When we think about the stomach, it is a vessel for sufficiency, adequacy, satisfaction, comfort, nourishment, provision, sharing, worth, and socializing. It is a container for abundance, and it tells us when we have had enough. The narrator's metaphors of breadwinning, providing and abundance—enough—all appear to say the exact same thing as his disease. This is the doorway to understanding not only the narrator's (my) disease, but also your own.

Exercise 6.1: Stop and notice

Objective: This exercise aims to enhance your self-awareness of your body through visualization and reflection on feelings related to various stomach-related metaphors. Instructions:

1. **Find a quiet space:** Choose a calm and comfortable environment where you can stand without distractions.

2. **Close your eyes:** Take a few deep breaths to center yourself. Inhale deeply through your nose, hold for a moment, and exhale slowly through your mouth.

3. **Visualize a hoop:** Imagine a large hoop laid out on the ground before you. This hoop represents an extension of your self-awareness. Alternatively, you can think of it as a smart piece of electronic wizardry that is capable of sensing your feelings.

4. **Step into the hoop:** Picture yourself standing in the middle of the hoop. Foster a sense of grounding and presence.

5. **Begin scanning your body:** Visualize the hoop rising slowly

from your toes, scanning your body. As it moves up your body, notice and acknowledge any sensations you feel including where in your body you feel them.

6. **Identify sensations:** As the hoop scans from your feet to the top of your head and back down, pay attention to any areas of your body that respond as you reflect on the following stomach-related metaphors:

    - **Sufficiency**: What sensations arise?
    - **Adequacy**: Notice any physical responses.
    - **Satisfaction**: Identify where you feel this in your body.
    - **Comfort**: Does this resonate with a particular area?
    - **Nourishment**: What feelings emerge?
    - **Provision**: Where do you sense this concept?
    - **Sharing**: Notice if any sensations arise.
    - **Worth**: Reflect on how this might feel in your body.
    - **Socializing**: What physical feelings does this bring up?
    - **Abundance**: Scan for any responses related to this idea.

7. **Explore your reactions**: If you feel discomfort, tension, or pain, acknowledge these feelings. Remember that there are no right or wrong responses—trust your experience.

8. **Personal reflection**: If you do not find a resonance with the metaphors, that is perfectly fine. Take a moment to explore any thoughts or feelings related to your own experiences with GERD. Write down any flashes of inspiration or insights that arise, noting what feels significant to you.

9. **Document your experience:** After completing the scan, take a few minutes to journal about your sensations and any insights gained from the exercise. Consider how these insights relate to your personal story.

10. **Revisit the exercise:** Return to this exercise periodically to deepen your understanding of the connection between your bodily sensations and your personal narratives.

Conclusion: This exercise invites you to engage with your body-mind, promoting awareness and understanding of your emotional and physical states. Over time, you may uncover deeper reflections that can enhance your overall well-being.

---

1. Proulx, T., Markman, K.D., & Lindberg, M.J., (2013). Introduction: The new science of meaning. In K.D. Markman, T. Proulx, & M.J. Lindberg (Eds.), The psychology of meaning (pp. 3-14). Washington, DC, USA; American Psychological Association.

2. Hollis, J., (2013). Theogonies and therapies: A Jungian perspective on humanity's dark side. In A.C. Bohart, B.S. Held, E. Mendelowitz, & K.J. Schneider (Eds.), Humanity's dark side: Evil, destructive experience, and psychotherapy (pp. 83-97). Washington, DC, USA; American Psychological Association.

3. Camus, A., (2004). The myth of Sisyphus. In G. Marino (Ed.), Basic writings of existentialism (pp. 441-492). New York, NY, USA; Random House. (Original work published 1942.)

Seven

The Five P's

The core lament

Psychotherapists and those in related fields are taught to evaluate a person's story to explain the core lament. This is the emotional pain that arises from an individual's past experiences, and their current identity and relationships. It embodies the sense of longing or nostalgia for what has been lost in one's life. Understanding a person's core lament can help the therapist address underlying issues and facilitate healing by allowing people to express their deepest feelings, uncovering the emotional wounds that may affect their current mental health and behavior. Working through this lament can lead to greater self-awareness, acceptance, and ultimately, personal growth.

Psychotherapists look for certain factors to find the core lament. In the same way that therapists use their knowledge of these factors to help people attain greater self-agency, we can apply these same factors to find and heal the core lament of physical disease.

Acknowledging these **Five P's** lends immediate insight when it comes to suffering because they build the understanding that all kinds of health problems are multifactorial. In other words, your GERD is explained by a number of factors that came together at the same time to create the perfect storm.

The Five P's are as follows:

- **Predisposing factors:** These are the factors that make us prone to illness, such as our family history, life events, and personal temperament.

- **Precipitating factors:** These are the factors that appear at the start of an illness and refer to a specific event or trigger that has an element of pain or suffering.

- **Presenting factors:** These are the obvious signs and symptoms that make up the somatic (body) story, and which are helpful in understanding somatic metaphor, which I will come to explain is the tip of the disease iceberg.

- **Perpetuating factors:** These are the factors that maintain the illness once it has become established and which are inevitably informed by our childhood experiences (e.g., a parent's behavior or anxiety) and our own feelings and thoughts around those experiences, as well as any associated behaviors.

- **Protective factors:** These are our strengths or sources of resilience that we can call on when we decide to take action to heal our illness and which help us to deal effectively with the stress in our lives.

My five P's

Returning to my own story of GERD as an example, we can identify each of these factors in turn.

Predisposing factors

Other than genetics (my mother also had GERD), the predisposing factors were being exposed as a child to my mother's financial problems, having a history of unfulfilling interpersonal relationships, and having a deep and unacknowledged feeling of inadequacy since childhood.

Precipitating factors

The triggers for my GERD were my wife becoming pregnant with our first child and about to quit her job, expectant fatherhood, starting a new business that was not yet providing enough income, and a tension around accepting my role as the family's chief and only breadwinner.

Presenting factors

When my GERD was diagnosed, my main complaints were heartburn, abdominal discomfort, bad breath, nighttime cough, and interrupted sleep. These symptoms are all explained in terms of acid injury to the esophagus, the tube that facilitates the passage of food into the stomach. More importantly, the origin of these symptoms in my stomach seemed to convey a symbolic meaning, as well as a medical one.

Perpetuating factors

These were a continued belief in my own inadequacy and of never having enough. Also, my regard of work as a need fulfillment for this inadequacy while overlooking past relational traumas. And finally, fulfilling my obligations to my family as their sole provider.

Protective factors

The things that helped me cope and eventually take action included my unwillingness to accept my doctor's view that I would always need to take omeprazole, as well as a strong curiosity about disease in general, a belief in a better world, and family support.

Of course, every story is different. And while it's useful to use someone else's story as a starting point, you will need to develop your own insights as you progress further into your story.

Exercise 7.1: Your five P's

Predisposing factors

Beginning with predisposing factors, what are the elements of your story that made you prone to GERD? Think of other people in your family with GERD: What other attributes might you share with them? What are the struggles that you have in common? I didn't just share GERD with my mother; I also acquired her beliefs about money, which were shaped by her own life experiences. We both navigated a number of traumas together that influenced my own perspective and journey. Here are some general examples to get you started:

- Genetics: I am my father's genes since he and his mother before him had GERD.

- Personality: I am a person who keeps things to themselves.

Precipitating factors

What life events provided the trigger for your GERD? If this isn't immediately obvious, have a think about what else was going on around the time your symptoms began. For me, it was my feelings and thoughts about my wife's pregnancy and the associated pressures for my business to succeed, and having to replace my wife as our breadwinner. This carried a lot of burden for me, as it had previously for my mother. Here are some general examples:

- Stress: I am stressed by situations in which I don't feel I have any control.

- Tiredness: I am tired of always being the responsible one.

- Financial: I am struggling to find abundance in my life.

Presenting factors

What are your symptoms? Notice how they might be explained in a symbolic sense based on their location. We know that stomach acid, when it enters the esophagus, can produce distressing symptoms in the chest, abdomen, mouth, and throat. Could the specific locations of your symptoms hold personal meaning to you? Heartburn, for example, might be more than a burning sensation in your chest; it could also describe a loss, or a current heartache in relationship.

Perpetuating factors

What factors do you believe are important in keeping your GERD going? Have a think of the areas of your life where your struggle is greatest. Is it a struggle for personal fulfillment, in your work and financial life, in your social life, or in your intimate relationships? What earlier events and core beliefs could this current struggle be related to? Here are some general examples:

- Work: I am dependent on my work as an expression of my status; work helps me to be more.

- Social: I am at a loss to find a true friend.

- Relationships: I am unseen/unheard in my family.

- Cultural: I am part of a wider cultural identity that includes my community, but I feel I don't belong.

- Diet: I am fond of [food] because it reminds me of...

- Exercise: I am reluctant to exercise less because exercise allows me to forget what happened when...

Protective factors

What protective factors do you currently have in your life? Knowing these will remind you why resolving GERD is important to you. Our protective factors are also a valuable source of support when the going gets a little tough.

Exercise 7.2: Preliminary journal jottings

Using the journal you are keeping, now is the time to write down some preliminary details of your story based on your five P's. In addition to each of the five factors, take a broader view of your ideas to uncover any ongoing emotional pain that connects these together. Think of past experiences and losses, as well as any current concerns.

These notes can be short, long, simple, complex; it is really up to you. You may choose to write in your own voice, but if your GERD started in childhood, consider writing in the voice of your child-self. Or, if your own voice feels too confronting, you could pretend that you are writing in the voice of a fictional character who also happens to have GERD. The key is whatever works best for you.

If what you write in your journal seems a little vague, that is okay. If it helps your story to emerge, why not do a drawing or a mind map of the things you want to say? You do not need to be an artist; use doodles and sketches, create a storyboard of ideas, add color. Stick figures are fine. Include old photos, newspaper clippings of the time, random jottings, anything that could be relevant as your story evolves. Here are some prompts:

- What was going on when your symptoms started?

- Where were you?

- What was happening in your different relationships?

- What were you working at or studying?

- What were the problems, challenges, concerns or neglects around the different aspects of your life?

- Did anything change (even if it seems insignificant), or did something remain the same?

- Did you experience any losses, big or small?

Eight

The Stomach as Metaphor

Somatic metaphor

Paul Simon once sang, "Why am I soft in the middle? The rest of my life is so hard."

The softness Simon referred to was a metaphor for an undesirable personality trait that draws on the imagery of a sagging belly. The use of such metaphors in storytelling is an efficient way to communicate complex ideas, including the feelings those ideas are founded on.

The language we use to describe ourselves, others and our experiences is filled with such metaphors that often trace to some part of the body. This embodied or somatic language (i.e., somatic metaphor) is an everyday phenomenon, yet we have lost any sense of the words as an expression of the body itself.

A useful analogy to understand the power of metaphor in the context of the body in general is the iceberg metaphor. We know when we see an iceberg, we are really looking at the top fraction floating above the waterline. What we don't see is the much greater fraction that remains hidden from our ordinary gaze beneath the ocean's surface.

We can think of the top fraction as the expression of our story, which becomes conscious to us when we recognize our own somatic metaphor. The remaining bulk is the unconscious expression whose hidden meaning is revealed through courageous self-exploration.

Here are some other general examples of somatic metaphor:

- Its beauty took my breath away.
- My heart skipped a beat.
- My nerves are on edge.
- Our victory was sweet.
- They're a pain in the neck.
- I put on a brave face.
- I can't stomach that.

Each metaphor gives us a snippet of something much larger, but this greater aspect is accessed only through deeper contemplation (see: *Unearthing the phenomenon*). The interpretation of the metaphor is of course subjective and dependent on one's own personal experiences.

Finding meaning from metaphor

Is it possible to find value or meaning beyond the ordinary gaze using the above examples of somatic metaphor? Well, yes. Let's look at the first statement, "Its beauty took my breath away."

If you retell a story of witnessing a whale breaching the ocean's surface, and realize during the retelling that you had been holding your breath in wonder when you saw the whale, then your story might hold special meaning to you. Even if you were not consciously aware of holding your breath when you saw the whale breach, your statement that "its beauty took my breath away" conveys an experience your body remembers.

When you recognize the link between the exact words of your story and its embodiment, you bring consciousness to the metaphor and the underlying meaning emerges.

Let's consider the statement, "I put on a brave face." If you developed a facial rash during a traumatic period in your life and you tell someone your method of coping was to "put on a brave face," then this too is potentially meaningful.

Or if you developed GERD at a time when your spouse was cheating on you, and your response to seeing someone else cheating on their spouse is to say, "I can't stomach that," then your words are potentially meaningful.

Trauma and metaphor

In their book *Trauma, Culture, and Metaphor: Pathways of Transformation and Integration*, Wilson and Lindy describe the metaphors we use to approach trauma.[1] Doctors might approach a person's trauma from a biological perspective using language that explores themes like abnormal physiology, medication and surgery. An anthropologist might approach trauma as a journey from the abyss, with exposure to peril, a commitment to an ideal greater than the self, and a difficult return home. The teacher might approach trauma as an exercise involving stuck-points and growth edges, requiring homework and making conclusions. The business person might approach trauma using themes of consumption and manufactured feelings.

With the disturbed "I Am," our expression of language and other symbols can reveal unexplored traumas from our past. The way it might work is like this:

First, when a person experiences trauma, the initial response of the wholeperson is unconscious and involves the bodymind finding ways to encode the traumatic experience for later recovery once immediate safety needs are met. Then, as the wholeperson lives and grows beyond the traumatic event, the unconscious maps any unresolved issues onto our spoken language and other important symbolic devices. These include non-verbal communication cues, personal mythologies, and the use of literature, art, dance and music as trauma outlets. Such symbols are a part of daily life and we use them as repositories of meaning until such time as we are ready to harvest that meaning. The wholeperson response to trauma is therefore adaptive, even if the illness or disturbed behavior that represents the trauma until it is resolved is maladaptive.

In a nutshell, we are continuously influenced by the metaphors in our lives. We don't speak these symbols so much as these symbols speak us. This is because metaphors have a way of holding the most truth in the least space. Unconsciously at least, we latch on to those metaphors that are efficient in communicating a particular meaning that is close to our own truth. As an example, let's further develop the analysis of my personal vignette from *Symptoms, story and meaning*.

The metaphor in my story

> I was thirty-two when I developed GERD. My symptoms began soon after my wife became pregnant with our first child at a time when I was struggling to get some financial ***momentum*** in my new business. Our child was planned, but I felt increasingly panicked as my wife's due date and work end date drew closer. We would no longer be able to rely on her as our main ***breadwinner***, and my business was not ***providing*** us with ***enough*** income to live on.

Viewing the stomach as a vessel for abundance, my use of the words "breadwinner," "providing" and "enough"—unconscious choices at the time—can be interpreted as somatic metaphors for feelings of insufficiency and inadequacy.

Considering what was going on in my life when my GERD symptoms first started, I experienced the loss of my wife's breadwinning support as a threat to our abundance. Moreover, having taken the baton from my wife, I doubted my own adequacy in the role of provider.

Hopefully it will now be obvious to you that there is a connection between the exact words we use in a literal sense and their often symbolic or hidden meaning. Words and phrases, such as regurgitate, give up, going down, tried everything, consume, move up, and store, are all potential metaphors for the stomach and therefore possible entry points into your own body story.

As a conduit between the mouth and stomach, the esophagus may be associated with words such as channel, hook-up, tie-up, attachment, connection, coupling, or transit. You can probably think of others too.

Stomach metaphors

Here are some stomach metaphors to get you thinking about your own GERD. These are separated into groups for easy exploration. If you come across any that resonate, think about any potential feelings, as well as personal meaning, that the metaphor holds. For example, if you resonate with "made me want to throw up," this might indicate feelings of disgust or rejection. If such feelings come up for you, think of a time in your life this relates to.

Physical, visceral or material metaphors

- Stomach tied in knots
- Butterflies in stomach
- Sick to the stomach
- Made stomach turn/churn
- Fire in the belly
- Made me want to throw up
- Cast iron/strong stomach

Emotional processing metaphors

- Can't take any/much more
- I've had enough
- Had a belly/guts full
- Difficult to stomach
- Hard to take

- Don't have the stomach
- Consumed by grief
- Swallowing your pride
- Taking it is a bitter pill
- Boiling with anger
- In a pit of despair
- Pain is too much

Self-worth, sufficiency and adequacy metaphors

- I'm not enough
- Not good enough
- Not worth enough
- Don't matter enough
- Doesn't hold its value
- Have nothing to offer
- Don't deserve anything
- Don't measure up
- Don't care enough
- I'll take what I can get

Intuition, defensiveness and associated feelings

- Had a gut feeling/instinct
- Pit of the stomach
- My stomach sank
- Had a sinking feeling
- Don't let your guard down
- Let my guard down

Emptiness, fullness and satiety metaphors

- Hungry for love
- Fed up with life
- Feeling empty/emptiness
- Stomach is a bottomless pit
- Got nothing more to give
- Full to burst
- Full of doubt
- Full of anger/grief
- I have nothing

Effort, opening, and work-related metaphors

- Worked guts off
- Busted my guts
- Spilled my guts
- Too many mouths to feed
- Too much on my plate

Power and control metaphors

- Don't get your hopes up
- Don't let us down
- Have cake and eat it too
- Got their just desserts
- Predatory appetite
- Eyes bigger than stomach
- Wolf in the belly
- Went belly up
- Called yellow belly
- No one backed me up
- Don't give it too much stock
- Expecting too much

Rumination and metaphors for thinking

- Chewing the cud/fat
- Navel gazing
- Gave food for thought

Containment metaphors

- Secrets that can't be spilt
- Can't hold (onto) anything
- Trying to keep things under control

Metaphors for scarcity and lack

- Don't earn enough
- Don't have enough
- Don't make enough
- Expecting too much

Submission metaphors

- It's settled then
- I give up

Although these metaphors can provide important clues about the meaning of your GERD, it is not essential to find a metaphor that exactly fits your particular circumstances. Rather, you are looking for an entry point into your story that allows you to align your physical symptoms (i.e., your stomach, esophagus and throat) with your story.

As I continued to reflect on the circumstances around my own GERD, the metaphor that seemed to hold the most truth in the least space was "I'm not enough." I knew this to be true because I felt the powerful resonance of these words within my stomach.

Exercise 8.1: Finding your GERD metaphor

Using the list of stomach metaphors above, speak aloud each metaphor in turn. As you sound out each metaphor, pay close attention to any bodily sensations. A strong bodily reaction to any given metaphor may suggest, at an unconscious level, you are resonant with its possible underlying meaning in your own story.

Enter your ideas into your journal.

---

1. Wilson, J. P., & Lindy, J. D., (eds.), (2013). Trauma, culture, and metaphor: Pathways of transformation and integration. New York, NY, USA; Routledge.

Nine

Your Story

Embracing your inner expert

All illnesses have a clear beginning marked by the first noticeable symptoms. After this initial occurrence, you may notice a certain rhythm to your symptoms, which can fluctuate hourly, daily, or even week to week. In other words, your GERD has new beginnings depending on when symptoms are present and when they are not.

The beginning, in whatever form it takes for you, is a great place to start unraveling your story. You can learn a lot about GERD based on what else was happening in your life when you first noticed symptoms, as well as what is currently occurring when symptoms worsen or improve.

As you begin to engage with your story, it is important to embrace your inner expert. Self-healing is an instinctive process that often requires paying attention to our inner dialogue and taking advantage of information that arrives in unexpected ways.

Possible entry points into your story—or some aspect of your story—include your dreams, conversations with others, news articles, music, or moments of quiet reflection.[1] The list is endless.

Be open to synchronicity, which involves finding meaning in separate events that, on the surface, may not appear to have a causal relationship. In other words, it's time to break away from any previously held beliefs you might have that reality is linear and confined to the physical limitations of space and time.

> *"Synchronicity is an inexplicable and profoundly meaningful coincidence that stirs the soul."*
>
> — Phil Cousineau

Think back to when your symptoms began. Do you remember *anything* significant happening in your life around that time? Where were you? What relationships were important then? Were there any problems in these areas?

Consider any significant changes, such as moving, changing schools, finding new friends, or starting a new relationship. What about losses, big or small? Were there any new births, illnesses, bereavements, unemployment, financial difficulties, memorable failures, work-related stressors, excessive responsibilities, or other burdens?

Here are a few tips as you start to reflect on your story:

- The key here is to note *anything*, whether it seems important or not.

- This is an exercise in recalling what you do remember, not in what you think you ought to remember.

- Things that come to mind quickly often turn out to be highly relevant.

- Avoid the temptation to rush through this process; take your time and find a comfortable spot to reflect quietly.

- Write down whatever comes to mind; your notes don't need to be in a form that makes sense to someone else.

The smorgasbord question

When I first started addressing my own GERD, I discovered that therapeutic insight came from asking the "smorgasbord question." This question shifts our focus from the illness itself to the important life events that occurred around the time our symptoms emerged.

Fortunately, the ordinary language we use to describe our life events is rich with information that can help us uncover meaning. Whether spoken or written, our language is always symbolic and can reference the healthy "I Am" or the disturbed "I Am" present in disease.

Based on the experiences of MindBody luminary, consultant immunologist, and psychotherapist Dr. Brian Broom, the smorgasbord question asks:

> What was the most interesting, memorable, significant, troublesome, difficult, problematic, hard, worrying, frustrating, or stressful thing or things happening in your life around the time your symptoms started? [2]

To begin exploring this question, take a moment for self-reflection using Exercise 9.1 below and see what comes up for you. Or, if you're really struggling, try the alternative Exercise 9.2.

Exercise 9.1: Smorgasbord self-reflection

Reflect on the life circumstances that accompanied the onset of your GERD symptoms.

Using the smorgasbord question, consider each prompt—starting with *interesting* and ending with *stressful*. You may find that one prompt stands out to you more than the others. If so, focus on that prompt and think about a specific life event that may need to come into your awareness.

Now, write down your thoughts without filtering, editing, or interpretation. Approach this as a *stream-of-consciousness* exercise where you write down *anything* that comes to mind.

It's beneficial to keep a journal, as there will be many useful opportunities for ongoing self-reflection and personal discovery.

Pushing through pain

If you feel distracted or want to end the exercise before finishing, there may be painful or scary emotions that you wish to avoid. If so, you have found your growth edge!

Remember: personal growth requires discomfort.

Instead of resisting discomfort, consider waiting a day before trying again. It's fine to engage gradually with your fear or pain rather than rushing. By pushing through the pain, you may trigger a memory or have a revealing dream.

You might ask someone close to you about what was happening in your life when your symptoms began. Listen carefully but be aware that this person may minimize their own feelings about significant life events.

Exercise 9.2: Solutions for smorgasbord strugglers

If you struggle to develop your response to the smorgasbord question, ask a trusted friend or family member to ask you the question. Then, without hesitation, say out loud the first thought that comes to mind. Avoid rehearsing possible responses beforehand or it will defeat the usefulness of the exercise.

Alternatively, have a conversation with the person about the time when you first developed GERD symptoms, using the individual prompts of the smorgasbord question to explore themes such as *difficult, memorable* or *troublesome*. Use your relationship with the other person to explore how you coped, what was hard for you at the time, and why it is important for you to find meaning now.

Remember, when exploring your story in this way, you are speaking from the whole of you. Your exact words are important so be sure to capture your words using a voice recorder or writing down what came up in conversation. It is always a good idea to keep a journal of your responses for later reflection.

Dealing with resistance

When answering the smorgasbord question, you may default to saying nothing was going on when you first developed GERD symptoms. Try to move beyond this temptation. Meaning enriches your life constantly. There is never truly nothing going on.

Here are some common reasons why people resist their stories and miss potential meaning.

Default positivity

Are you habitually positive, regardless of your actual circumstances?

From a young age we often learn to avoid the reality of our significant emotions (see: *We are trained not to feel*.) This conditioning leads us to be overly positive no matter what we actually feel.

This is no better demonstrated than in the world of social media where some influencers lie routinely to prove the merits of their fake "lives less ordinary."

If you struggle with the smorgasbord question because you believe you need to overlook a harsher reality in order to maintain a veneer of optimism, it is time to get real and be kind to yourself. Personal growth does not happen because we wear a mask of positivity but because we are ready to embrace our shadow and invite the rich meaning that this unexplored aspect of self wants to reveal.

Fear of difficult things

Do you have any anxiety or fear around thinking and saying something difficult?

When facing any life-threatening situation, our instincts guide us to counter the threat using flight, fight or freeze strategies. This is a healthy fear response intended to get us away from the threat to our immediate safety. But when a fear stimulus is more nuanced and ongoing, the same strategies are unhelpful and unhealthy, yet often remain part of our adaptive response to fear.

In Western cultures, we are conditioned to resist anything that causes discomfort. Fear by its very nature is uncomfortable. It is also unavoidable, but when it happens we try to put distance between ourselves and it. Instead of feeling the fear, we might lash out in anger, run away from the problem, or bury it in the body in the form of hives, high blood pressure, or some other physical illness. As long as we resist our fears, they have a dark and painful hold over us.

How we react to fear may be innately driven, but how we choose to act in response to fear is a choice. If we no longer want fear to control our lives, rather than avoiding it we need to *lean* into it. By lean, I mean we must feel the fear in its fullness, allowing it to be experienced in the body, observing it as an impartial onlooker would even renaming it non-judgmentally, for example as "this feeling in my chest." As you experience fear in this conscious and intentional way, you may find that your fear begins to fade without needing to push it away.

Resisting connections between symptoms and events

Have you noticed a connection between your GERD and certain life events?

We often ignore significant feelings while focusing on symptoms in the belief—or hope—that they are fixable.

With our symptoms top-of-mind and feelings ignored, the life events that evoke dynamic feelings remain unprocessed and move quickly into the past. It does not help that we are often taught to view ourselves as victims of circumstance who simply react to life's events, rather than individuals who can steer our own course.

Symptoms emerge from the whole "I Am" and not merely through the physical dimension of personhood. When we use conscious intention to recognize the connections between GERD and story, we create the conditions for our reconnection and recovery.

Recalling the iceberg analogy, the tip of the iceberg is our story expressed through somatic metaphor; the remaining bulk is the unconscious expression or hidden meaning. Just *knowing* about a connection can be healing. This is because we begin using the energy we convert ordinarily into symptoms for a healthier purpose. Our disease-messenger has gained our attention and our

GERD symptoms are no longer needed! Learn to trust your feelings and get comfortable exploring them, along with your story around key life events.

Looking for catastrophes when mishaps will suffice

Do you tend to catastrophize, thinking things are or will end up worse than your actual circumstances warrant?

Major crises such as a loved one's death, a breakup, job loss, or other significant event occur to all of us, but your story does not have to be about any of these things. It could be about the arrival of a new sibling, a new friendship, shifting home or school, or any number of different events or discoveries.

Remember, your response to the smorgasbord question depends on what you allow to come to the surface. It is important that you do not dismiss any life event as unimportant or trivial. If a detail comes to you, treat it with curiosity rather than contempt. It might lead you somewhere important.

---

1. Feinstein, D., & Krippner, S., (2008). Personal mythology: Using ritual, dreams, and imagination to discover your inner story. Santa Rosa, CA, USA; Energy Psychology Press/Elite Books.

2. Broom, B., (2007). Meaning-*full* disease: How personal experience and meanings cause and maintain physical illness. Oxfordshire, UK; Routledge.

TEN

Identifying Specific Memories

Memories and metaphor

As I have mentioned, finding meaning from your GERD requires endeavor and detour. Metaphor offers an entry point into our body story, but this is just the tip of the iceberg. The real value resides with further evaluation of the unconscious aspects of our story and is vital to healing GERD.

When uncovering the metaphor "I'm not enough," I had been reflecting on important relationships when I was a child. This necessarily brought up certain memories, some of them quite painful. It is intriguing how patterns of experience recur habitually in our lives, highlighting the importance of examining these patterns through our memories. For instance, whereas my wife had been the main breadwinner when my business was taking flight, my mother held that role in my childhood home following my parents' divorce.

While thinking about this pattern involving important women in my life as the main breadwinners, I recalled a miserable Saturday morning when I was ten years old. My football team had just lost our game and my mood was as frosty as the day. Driving home afterwards, my mother stopped on the side of the road and burst into tears. I thought my irritability had gotten to her, but it was her own distress, and it would have far worse consequences than a lost football game.

Coaxing my mother into sharing her troubles, I learned that her bank was threatening to foreclose on our home mortgage due to difficulties in keeping up with the loan repayments. My stomach sank. There was already precious little security in my life and now we were about to lose our home.

I told my mother that I would help her with the loan by getting a newspaper delivery job. I was not expecting her to laugh at me! She was not trying to be mean, but her insensitivity to my sincere offer added more than a drop of fuel to an already burgeoning belief in my own inadequacy. From that experience I also learned that I would never be able to earn enough, failing to consider that I was just a kid and newspaper delivery jobs paid for candy, not home loans.

As an adult, my reflections of that day helped uncover the underlying feeling in my stomach that "I'm not enough." I continued to explore the themes from my childhood that appeared to fit my body story, ultimately relating these themes to becoming my family's breadwinner and the onset of GERD. The feelings of inadequacy and insufficiency that I felt in my stomach as a child were now manifesting as a disease of the stomach in my adulthood.

As I got deeper into the different levels of this story, my current worries about financial security morphed into the more meaningful realization that I lacked nourishment and emotional security in key childhood relationships. I uncovered a variation of the previous metaphor, "I never have enough."

Exploring these relationships through regular self-reflection provided the tipping point for my GERD symptoms. As I evaluated these relationships within the context of the core beliefs of "I'm not enough" and "I never have enough," I realized I had been holding on to grief and shame. In the section on *Working with feelings*, I show you how to address these and other significant feelings, which are an inevitable aspect of any disease.

In 2015, I presented my experiences of resolving GERD, along with James' story, as a case series in the peer-reviewed journal *Energy Psychology: Theory, Research, and Treatment*.[1] I wrote my "disease emerged as a struggle with self against a backdrop of unfulfilling interpersonal relationships in childhood."

This reference to fulfillment turned out to be a further unconscious expression of my GERD that proved helpful when I experienced a brief relapse some years after the article's publication. It was almost as if I had written a note to my future self to dig a little deeper. Instead of having GERD for five years this second time round, my symptoms lasted just two days!

Linking GERD with specific memories

It is common during routine self-reflection to recall specific memories of another time. Most often these memories distract us from whatever thoughts we had when the memory came up. Our mind is a wanderer and requires we take a disciplined approach in order to make conscious linkages between a problem we are ruminating on and the recall of a specific earlier memory.

It is plausible that our mind wanders in this way due to our early life conditioning, which teaches us that our lives are random and meaningless, and that we must avoid our significant feelings for the discomfort they cause. A wandering and easily distracted mind appears to be the consequence!

So when self-reflecting on your GERD, it is important that when you do recall a specific memory to treat its recall as meaningful, however unrelated your memory may seem. In a way, you are retraining your bodymind to expect to make meaningful linkages between a current challenge and earlier life events. Let your instincts guide you in this. Make a note of each memory in a journal so you can come back to them again and again if need be.

You do not need to have a conscious memory of a particular life event in order to take advantage of the possibilities for healing. When I had exhausted all options for resolving trichotillomania, I recalled my mother telling me once that as a 10-month old infant, I banged my head deliberately and repeatedly against the wall.

This reported episode along with my imagination proved to be the opening I needed to finally overcome this distressing impulse control disorder.

Without a conscious memory of banging my head against the wall, I imagined what that would have been like for 10-month old me. I asked myself important questions, such as what experiences would prompt a child of just 10 months to self-harm? What was my living situation like? What were my relationships with family members like? What sort of relationship did I have with my primary attachment, my mother? (See: *Feelings as connection*.)

Asking these questions took me on an important journey of self-discovery. Allowing my imagination to roam, I intuited that at 10 months old I needed to feel pain in order to overcome the numbness of not being met in relationship.

This conclusion helped me to cross a threshold beyond which I no longer felt the irrepressible urge to pull out my hair. It all happened in a moment that took 28 years to arrive. But the healing was immediate and profound.

So when you are exploring any life events for their possible relationship to your GERD, allow *anything* that comes into your consciousness. Although we do not have any conscious recall of much of our life, the bodymind remembers. We can therefore make use of any information that comes to us to unlock and process the traumas trapped in our personal and embodied histories.

As you look deeper into your own story for specific memories that are resonant with your GERD, there are two ideas that may assist your endeavor and detour. The first of these is phenomenology and the second is hermeneutics. Both ideas have philosophical origins and are most often dealt with together. For simplicity, I have split the two ideas into their own chapters, with the first of these *Unearthing the phenomen*on and the second *Hermes, the messenger*.

Exercise 10.1: The transformative powers of journaling

Many people find that hand writing their thoughts and experiences has a unique power and resonance in the healing process. While putting pen to paper may hold particular significance for some, different mediums can equally facilitate exploration and expression for people who prefer a fresh avenue for self-discovery.

If this sounds like you, consider making audio recordings, where you speak your thoughts aloud, allowing your emotions and reflections to flow in a more spontaneous and personal way. You might transcribe these recordings later to capture your words in writing.

Alternatively, creating short videos of yourself speaking to the camera can provide a visual and dynamic way to connect with your feelings, enabling you to engage with your body language as you express your story.

Beyond these options, you could explore creative outlets like drawing or doodling to represent your feelings visually, or engaging in body movement to express and release emotions physically.

All these methods—whether auditory, visual, or kinesthetic—can enrich your understanding of your GERD journey. While reflecting on your experiences, let your chosen medium *speak* for you.

As you write or record the details of your GERD story, consider the following prompts related to emotionally difficult life situations that may have a resonance with your own experiences. Think of when your symptoms first started, and considering each of the prompts for possible alignment, allow your thoughts and feelings to emerge:

1. **Career pressure**: Think about a time when you faced significant pressure at work or school; perhaps a demanding project or an imminent deadline. How did this stress impact your well-being?

2. **Major life changes**: Reflect on a significant transition, such as moving to a new place, changing jobs, or ending a relationship. What feelings arose, and how did they manifest in your body?

3. **Family dynamics**: Consider moments of tension within your family, such as conflicts during holiday gatherings or challenges surrounding caregiving responsibilities. How did these experiences affect your emotional state and physical health?

4. **Loss or grief**: Recall a time when you experienced a significant loss, whether it was the death of a loved one or the end of an important relationship. How did your body respond to the grief during that period?

5. **Social status and comparison**: Write about experiences where you felt inadequate due to comparing yourself to others, whether in social situations, academic settings, or on social media. How did these feelings of

inadequacy manifest physically?

6. **Unmet expectations**: Reflect on situations where you felt you had fallen short of expectations—either your own or those of others. How did this sense of failure impact your emotional health?

7. **Fear of judgment**: Think about moments where you felt fearful of being judged or criticized by others. Did this fear create tension or discomfort in your body?

8. **Financial insecurity**: Recall times when you were worried about finances, whether due to job loss, unexpected expenses, or instability. How did this financial anxiety play into your overall sense of security and well-being?

9. **Isolation and loneliness**: Consider experiences where you felt isolated or disconnected from those around you. How did feelings of loneliness influence your mental and physical state during those times?

10. **Conflict with authority**: Reflect on instances where you found yourself in conflict with authority figures, such as a boss, teacher, or parent. How did these power dynamics affect your stress levels and physical symptoms?

11. **Overwhelming responsibilities**: Write about times when you felt burdened by excessive responsibilities—either at work, home, or in your social life. How did this overwhelm impact your emotional and physical well-being?

12. **Unresolved childhood feelings**: Consider any lingering emotions from childhood, such as feeling misunderstood or neglected. How might these unresolved feelings be echoing your present circumstances?

13. **Struggles with intimacy**: Reflect on difficulties in establishing or maintaining intimate relationships. Did these struggles create emotional tension that manifests in your body?

14. **Boundaries ignored or set**: Reflect on a moment when you were asked to do something important, or when you were specifically asked not to do something. How did that impact you?

15. **Acknowledgment and validation**: Reflect on moments when you felt unrecognized or unappreciated. How did this influence your sense of self-worth? Or recall something someone said to you that lingered in your mind. How was your self-perception impacted?

16. **Silence and recognition**: Reflect on times when someone didn't say something you needed to hear. How did that unspoken acknowledgment affect you?

17. **Dependency in relationships:** Consider instances where someone depended on you for support or you depended on someone else for support. Did that reliance create any feelings of vulnerability or fear?

18. **Feelings of exclusion**: Think back to a time you felt bored, excluded, overwhelmed in a social setting. What were the circumstances surrounding those feelings?

You can also journal about any new beginnings of your symptoms, rather than their original onset. The same prompts apply as before, only perhaps the events in question will be fresher in your mind. This is not an exhaustive list of prompts; you can come up with your own ideas. Remember not to judge possible events as being important or unimportant.

1. Christian, H.B., (2015). Subjective dimensions of meaning in the clinical encounter: Unifying personhood and disease. *Energy Psychology: Theory, Research and Treatment*, 7(1): 30–38.

ELEVEN

Unearthing the Phenomenon

Moving below our surface-level observations

The case studies I've presented involving James' cancer and my own GERD show how we can move away from our ordinary focus on symptoms toward the partial meaning of somatic metaphor—the tip of the iceberg. This in turn takes us beneath the surface waves of experience to the deeper phenomenon of our meaningful disease.[1] As mentioned before, when this meaning arrives, it is uniquely your own. It is not negotiated like a diagnosis, and you alone will be aware of its resonance in your body. Deeper feelings may emerge as you journey further into your story.

One way to think of this deep inward journey toward meaning is that it is like unearthing an experience for which we have no real appreciation or understanding until we bring it to consciousness. This immediately begs the question, How do we look for something—let alone find it—when we don't know what we are looking for?

The field of phenomenology deals effectively with this problem. Based on an ancient Greek root meaning *to appear*, a phenomenon is something that shows itself or makes itself manifest. The field of phenomenology emerged early last century as a branch of philosophy whose source of meaning and value is our own lived experience.

In his book, *Being and Time*, Martin Heidegger emphasized that a person's lived experience is meaningful and therefore a way to understand the subjective nature of our existence.[2] Heidegger's ideas, along with the work of other phenomenologists, have positively influenced modern healthcare practice, including in the areas of patient-centered care, qualitative research, mental health, and end-of-life care. Phenomenology invites a deeper engagement with the complexities of human experience, and enriches healthcare practice by providing more meaningful support for patients.

The appearance of phenomena

We can use phenomenology to describe our conscious experiences when interacting with the objects of our direct experience.[3] An example is the dinner table, which to look upon is not the same as the experience of eating with family at the dinner table. To recognize an object as a dinner table is only ever the appearance of a deeper phenomenon that requires us to experience the dinner table from our own practical, lived experience.

The appearance then is the phenomenon announcing itself "through something which does not show itself."[4] To *know* the phenomenon of your family dinner table, you first have to consider your experiences. This could involve *experiencing* the table during family rituals, social gatherings, or any other context in which the table appears to you, the experiencer. The phenomenon is never its appearance for it remains hidden from our ordinary gaze.

The semblance of phenomena

Sometimes we can be fooled into thinking we know the phenomenon of our lived experience when in fact we have stumbled onto the semblance of the phenomenon. For example, I can recall several different experiences at the family dinner table as a young child. There was a superficial enjoyment that accompanied my experiences so I could conclude that the family dinner table was a symbol for togetherness.

But when I consider these experiences more deeply, they reveal a darker complexity, suggesting that any superficial enjoyment was an illusion of harmony based on social obligation. The semblance then is when the phenomenon of our lived experience shows itself "as something which it is not." To use Heidegger's ideas, it is illusion and distortion.

Unearthing the phenomenon

Continuing with this personal example, my deeper reflections around childhood mealtimes uncovered a lack of genuine warmth and intimacy. I learned to shovel food down my throat to quickly finish the meal, rather than appreciate the nuances of flavor and the effort my mother expended in preparing our family dinners. I learned to avoid eye contact with my father at certain times. And I learned about the importance of pleasing others in order to avoid their displeasure, even if that meant ignoring my own needs.

The phenomenon of the dinner table from my lived experience was not as a space for togetherness (the semblance). It was a space defined by tacit expectations, unexpressed feelings, masked struggles, and unexamined histories.

The phenomenon of GERD

We can use the same understanding to help unearth the phenomenon of our GERD. A good starting point is our symptoms, which we must address if only to answer the smorgasbord question we considered in *Your story*.

Symptoms are clearly important, but focusing on these is no different to seeing a dinner table and thinking we know everything there is to know about it without factoring in our subjective lived experience. Our symptoms then are only ever the appearance of the phenomenon. Thought of in this way, our GERD symptoms are alerting us to the phenomenon, but are not themselves the phenomenon.

This is why we can treat symptoms endlessly—as biomedicine seeks to do—yet they persist and even progress over time. To fully experience the phenomenon of GERD and not just its appearance, we need to look deeper within.

Remember: *The phenomenon of your GERD announces itself through something which does not show itself.*

As we begin to harvest the meaning of GERD using a meaning-based story approach, we move closer to the phenomenon. You may already have a sense of this meaning based on your own reflections from previous chapters. You may have felt a lessening or change in quality of your symptoms as a result. Nevertheless, your GERD may remain unresolved.

When we experience a small taste of freedom from symptoms or subtle changes in symptom quality and occurrence, this might be the *semblance* of the phenomenon. So do not be discouraged if your GERD persists after a period of feeling better. On the contrary, simply noticing any changes in symptom frequency and/or quality indicates that you are becoming more mindful of your GERD. This mindfulness is helpful in heeding the lessons and moving more deeply into your story where the phenomenon waits to be unearthed.

Remember: *The semblance of the phenomenon occurs when the phenomenon shows itself as something which it is not.*

A case example

Maria (not her real name) is a 42-year old high school English teacher who enjoys gardening and participating in local theater productions. She is married with two children. She consults her primary care doctor for a persistent nighttime cough, alongside frequent episodes of heartburn and a sour taste after meals. Her symptoms have persisted for about four months, impacting her sleep quality and ability to concentrate at work. Maria tells her doctor that she sips water to "settle" her nighttime cough. She hopes treatment will "settle down" her symptoms and restore her sleep quality and productivity at work. After running some tests, Maria's doctor makes a GERD diagnosis and she is prescribed medication that gives her some relief.

The appearance of the phenomenon

Maria's symptoms of nighttime cough, disturbed sleep, frequent heartburn, sour taste after eating and difficulty concentrating are the phenomenon of her GERD announcing itself through something which does not show itself.

The Semblance of the Phenomenon

Maria's repetition of the word "settle" is potentially meaningful for the context in which she uses it. It is a somatic metaphor that potentially maps what appears to be a need for control in her life onto her stomach. As such, it provides an entry point into the deeper meaning of her story. When asked what else in her life other than her symptoms she wants to settle down, Maria replies, "I suppose things are a bit hectic at home and at work at the moment. It'd be nice if I didn't have so much stress in my life."

The question has the intended effect of drawing Maria away from her symptoms and getting her to look more deeply at her story. We determine that she was preparing for a teaching evaluation at work, while managing a hectic schedule filled with lesson plans, grading assignments, the needs of her two young children, and supporting her husband during a difficult time in his career. After making the connection between her symptoms and her need for things at work and home to settle down, Maria experiences an improvement in her GERD. However, this period of remission doesn't last.

This is the semblance of Maria's phenomenon of GERD, which shows itself as something which it is not.

The actual phenomenon

When Maria is pressed to find a deeper connection with her story, she begins to describe an earlier life experience that appears to scaffold to her present lived experience of needing things to be settled. In her teenage years, Maria's parents went through a tumultuous divorce marked by frequent arguments and emotional tension at home. She often found herself wishing for peace amidst the chaos, and on several occasions, she overheard her mother say they needed to "settle everything" for the sake of the family's happiness. Despite these attempts, for a long time issues remained unresolved, with Maria herself feeling deeply "unsettled," helpless, anxious and caught in the middle of her parents' dispute.

When asked how she coped, Maria said she became quite rebellious in her late teens, with the experience leaving her with "a sour taste in my mouth."

As an adult, Maria's need for peace stemmed from this formative life experience, influencing her desire for harmony and stability in her career and family life. Given the opportunity to properly process this experience, Maria's symptoms rapidly improved and she is now free of GERD. She maintains a better life balance through increased participation in gardening and theatre, and has learned to relax more during the day rather than accumulate tension that previously manifested during the night.

When the going gets tough

At this point, your journal is becoming a valuable source of potential insight and meaning. Remember to review your entries regularly to see if new understanding emerges from the stories you have recorded. Your patience and perseverance will be rewarded because the phenomenon of your GERD wants to be revealed! But coming to meaning is a journey and cannot be rushed.

If you are having difficulties getting to the deeper layers of your story, there could be a couple of possible reasons that may make it difficult to experience the fullness of the phenomenon that is your GERD. Maybe you have:

- Experienced some of the fullness of the phenomenon, but are having difficulties holding the significant feelings that accompany it. You may be highly defended against the phenomenon and these defenses become more engaged the closer you get to it.

- Found partial meaning, which has brought a change in your symptom frequency and/or quality, but the deeper meaning is yet to emerge. You may be searching for a *sameness* or a phenomenon with an everyday quality to it when what your story needs is to go beyond everyday consciousness to meet the unfamiliar and novel that we find when we are focused and curious.

Again, your patience and perseverance are key when working through such issues. A later section of the book is dedicated to *Working with feelings*, as well as the defenses that we use unconsciously to avoid our significant feelings, which can be uncomfortable and upsetting. Meanwhile, the remainder of this section looks at other ways into our story and the meaning to be found as we become more attuned to our bodyminds. Before moving to the next chapter, try the exercise below.

Exercise 11.1: Unearthing the Phenomenon of your GERD through mindful awareness

Objective: To cultivate awareness of GERD symptoms, explore their meanings, and uncover insights related to your discomfort.

Note: This exercise is best done when you are experiencing a flare in your symptoms.

1. **Settle into a comfortable posture:** Find a comfortable seated position that allows you to relax and focus. Ensure you are in a quiet environment where you won't be disturbed.

2. **Notice where your consciousness is normally directed:** Take a moment to notice that your consciousness is always directed toward something. Where does your attention normally go? Sometimes this is your thoughts, much less commonly your embodied sensations and emotions, and most often an activity you are performing. How true is this for you?

3. **Direct your attention to your GERD symptoms:** Shift your consciousness to your GERD and specifically wherever you feel symptoms in your body. Acknowledge these symptoms.

4. **Release judgment:** Let go of any need to label your symptoms as good or bad. Remember, they simply are. Avoid thoughts that categorize your symptoms as painful or unpleasant; these labels are not helpful for this exercise.

5. **Lean more deeply into your discomfort:** Immerse yourself

in the experience of your symptoms. Give them your full attention—observe what arises without distraction.

6. **Explore the connection:** As you focus all your attention on your symptoms, notice how the lines between your symptoms and yourself begin to blur. Understand that your GERD is part of your experience—not separate from you.

7. **Ask reflective questions:** Begin to delve into the meaning behind your symptoms by asking yourself:

    ○ "What message is my GERD attempting to send me?"

    ○ "How does expressing this disease serve me?"

    ○ "What rewards do I receive from having this disease?"

    ○ "What limiting belief helps to sustain this disease?"

    ○ "What would happen if I were to let go of this disease and gain freedom from it?"

8. **Journal your insights:** When you feel ready, journal any insights that emerged during your reflection. Document the messages you received and how they might influence your understanding of your GERD.

9. **Conclude the exercise:** Take a few deep breaths to ground yourself. Gently transition back to your regular activities, carrying any insights forward into your day.

---

1. Broom, B., (2007). Meaning-*full* disease: How personal experience and meanings cause and maintain physical illness. Oxfordshire, UK; Routledge.

2. Heidegger, M., (1962). Being and Time. In: J. Macquarrie, & E. Robinson, (Trans.), New York, NY, USA; Harper & Row.

3. To quote the theoretical physicist, Richard Feynman, "You can know the name of...[a] bird in all the languages of the world, but when you're finished, you'll know absolutely nothing whatever about the bird. You'll only know about humans in different places, and what they call the bird. So let's look at the bird and see what it's doing—that's what counts."

4. Heidegger, M., (1962). Being and Time. In: J. Macquarrie, & E. Robinson, (Trans.), New York, NY, USA; Harper & Row.

TWELVE

Hermes, the Messenger

Another way into the depths of the GERD iceberg is through hermeneutics. Named after Hermes who was messenger to the gods of Olympus, hermeneutics offers a unique pathway to healing for people struggling with GERD. As for the previous chapter that introduced phenomenology, hermeneutic inquiry is useful for exploring your personal narrative and its deeper meanings. Originally a branch of knowledge applied to the interpretation of literary texts, hermeneutics is especially useful when you are reflecting on your journal entries to find hidden meaning.

In addition to its uses in journaling, we can also apply the hermeneutic lens to other symbolic devices in order to bring meaning to light. Finding meaning from somatic metaphor, for example, is a form of hermeneutic interpretation since it deals with the hidden or embodied meaning in language. All forms of creativity are potential repositories of meaning, including creativity embedded in verbal and non-verbal communication, as well as written communication. Depending on the creativity that most resonates with you, the communication of meaning related to your own GERD may come from art, ceremony, crafts, dance, drama, music, mythology, or any number of endeavors.

As for the last chapter on *Unearthing the phenomenon*, the meaning found through interpreting a symbol does not arrive via a direct route. Rather, meaning-making requires a detour through the hermeneutic lens we choose (or which chooses us).

Again, the practice of hermeneutics requires movement beyond the surface level of physical discomfort to uncover insights related to any underlying emotional, psychological and social factors that may contribute to your GERD. You might reflect on your metaphor, a memory you wrote down in words, a painting you painted or a dance you performed to express your feelings. In the same way that these creative forms are aspects of your "I Am," you may find something meaningful that is relevant to the disturbed "I Am" of your GERD.

By applying hermeneutic methods, the healing journey becomes an integrative experience that fosters self-awareness and empowers you to make meaningful connections to further explore. If, despite this meaning, you remain stuck in your symptoms, it is natural to feel disheartened. The temptation is to want to reach the end of your journey with GERD, and quickly! But true hermeneutic interpretation is a cyclical process and does not succumb to linear thinking. There is no beginning or end within the *hermeneutic circle*.

The hermeneutic circle in a nutshell

As shown in the figure below, our entry point into the hermeneutic circle is the need to find meaning, such as from an event or experience. We can think of this as "the part" or an abstraction of the whole. In the next stage of hermeneutic interpretation, we use a symbolic device of our choosing to explore possible meaning. This could be a journal, a drawing, a previously identified somatic metaphor, music, or something else that resonates with you.

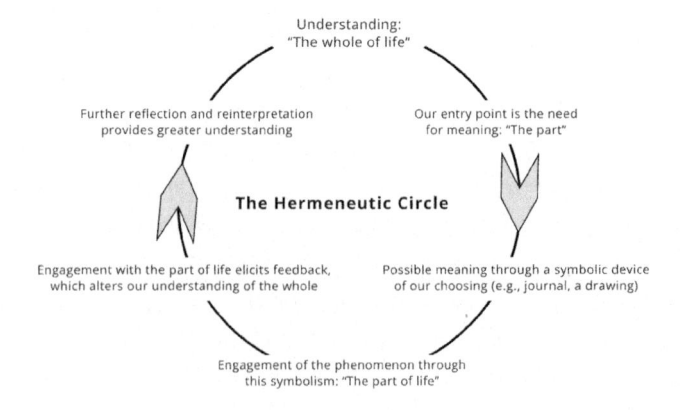

Figure 12.1: *Interpretation of a symbolic device for possible meaning using the hermeneutic circle.*

Next, we use our chosen symbolic device to uncover or engage with the phenomenon that we wish to interpret. This is where you can apply your understanding of phenomenology to look for the meaning in your own lived experience of GERD. The part becomes "the part of life." As we mindfully engage with the phenomenon and reflect on its personal meaning, our continued immersion in this process helps us to elicit feedback. This in turn alters our understanding of the whole.

Subsequent reinterpretation of this challenge to our understanding leads to greater self-awareness. Finally, heightened self-awareness contributes to our "whole of life" understanding, not only of our GERD, but also of our wholeperson. You are encouraged to continue to engage with this symbolic device through which to explore your GERD. In this way, new meaning may emerge from an ongoing cycle of self-reflection, reinterpretation and evolving self-awareness. It is the nature of hermeneutics to transport us through an endless loop of enlivenment.

The hermeneutic circle: The entry point

When entering the hermeneutic circle, you have options as to where to start. You could begin with the time in your life when you first noticed GERD symptoms. You could take a whole-of-disease approach where you engage with your chosen symbolic apparatus to explore your current symptoms. Or you could take a single aspect of your story or a specific memory.

Whichever you choose, the hermeneutic process is flexible enough to meet you at your point of readiness. Think of it like a holographic image: you can slice through such an image to create a series of parts, any of which can be used to recreate the whole. But instead of looking for sameness or the familiar, you are looking for novelty and new understanding.

You can also use the hermeneutic process to recover old ground with the intention of re-entering the circle to gain fresh insight. Hermeneutics often reveals the value of returning to previously chartered territory. For example, think of a time when a friend started to repeat a story they'd previously told you. Imagine that instead of tuning out or telling them that you'd already heard that particular story, you chose to listen attentively. Perhaps you noticed how their story was more nuanced or different in some way, whether because a new aspect of the story emerged or the way they told the story had changed and the feeling with it.

The hermeneutic circle: Symbolism

As we have discussed, all forms of creativity are potential repositories of meaning. But unless we know *how* to look, such meaning is difficult to find. That is where symbolism comes into its own. Written text, such as from journaling, is one example of how we use symbols to communicate information.

As long as you as the writer *and* reader of your journal understand the symbols of the text and the way you have used them, then in most cases the information received is the same as the information encoded or sent. But what if you don't understand something you were attempting to communicate earlier? What happens if your journal entry makes about as much sense to you as hieroglyphics? Or what if your video journal became corrupted in part, leaving the bulk of your entry unable to be decoded in a conventional way?

Fortunately, any work we do with the symbols of our GERD is naturally an intuitive process. As such, we are not reliant on logic, objectivity or information that arrives linearly and only via the five special senses.

Intuition is the sudden and unexpected arrival of *knowing* without needing to question or understand how the knowledge comes to us. It is a wholeperson experience, as in "I had a gut feeling." Accordingly, this knowing works seamlessly with creativity, which is a whole-of-life process that holds a special purpose or joy for each of us. As a writer must write, so too a sculptor must sculpt, a painter must paint, and a video blogger must vlog. How, what, when, where and why the writer, sculptor, painter or vlogger creates is an intuitive process.

Symbols, in contrast to the creativity that bears them, are an abstraction of the whole. Symbols work well with our intuition in that they are also an aspect in which the whole meaning is encoded, much like a hologram. Because of this, we do not need to be able to *see* the whole to be able to work with the whole.

Now suppose you encoded another meaning in your journal that was unconscious to you at the time of writing. Is it possible that you may identify this unconscious meaning when you later reflect on earlier journal entries?

Let me share a personal anecdote, which I mentioned earlier in the chapter *Identifying specific memories*. You'll recall that I presented my experiences of resolving GERD in a peer-reviewed journal article.[1] At the time, I wrote that my "disease emerged as a struggle with self against a backdrop of unfulfilling interpersonal relationships in childhood." When I used the word "unfulfilling," I was being literal in my efforts to efficiently describe my childhood dynamics. But at the time of writing, I was unconscious to this specific use of metaphor and its relevance to my GERD. When my symptoms returned some years after publishing the article, I had an intuitive prod to return to that article. Upon reviewing my earlier words, I immediately spotted the metaphor and applied its meaning to my current symptoms, which quickly resolved while processing this deeper aspect of my story.

The message here is that we often encode our symbols unconsciously, providing a clear reason for returning to our reflections to unearth further meaning.

The hermeneutic circle: Eliciting feedback

Whenever we use hermeneutics to engage with the phenomenon, our intuition serves as feedback, providing clues as to what needs to happen next. For example, if you have been journaling about relationships that seem to influence your GERD symptoms and suddenly recall a specific memory, then that intuitive feedback is the clue to where to go next.

Here's a case example:

Amar had been grappling with adult-onset GERD for years, but was encouraged recently to use a hermeneutic approach to seek meaning from his experience. During a moment's reflection, he recalled a time when his mother had shared a story of his struggles as an infant with reflux. His symptoms—most noticeably regurgitation—began soon after he was weaned from breastfeeding at three months old and ended when he came off infant formula.

Initially, Amar believed this recall was insignificant, but he held onto it in the belief that it could yet reveal insights.

Much as Amar preferred to push aside such "insignificant" details, you too might feel ambivalent about your GERD. Yet, when your symptoms or a symbolic memory do reclaim your attention, look to your environment for new symbols or cues that offer motivation. Reflect on this feedback in the moment, if you can, and let it guide your next steps.

Later, while revisiting his journal, Amar noticed a book on his desk that immediately captured his attention: "Born a Crime." This title resonated deeply, sparking further reflection.

The hermeneutic circle: Reinterpretation

Whenever we are stuck with the feedback that we do receive from our GERD story, this is always an opportunity to reinterpret our findings. Any stalled feedback is akin to recognizing the appearance, or more likely the semblance, of the phenomenon, with the continued challenge being to recognize the phenomenon itself. It may seem endless or possibly even futile, but again perseverance is key: There is no meaning without endeavor and detour.

This is an appropriate juncture to continue with Amar's story:

When Amar next reflected on his GERD, another memory surfaced; this time of his mother telling him that his constant regurgitation of the infant formula she fed him left him distressed and his father angry. This led to a further memory in which his actions on a losing sports team provoked his father's stern rebuke and the statement that "You don't have the fire in your belly, you need to toughen up!"

When Amar chose to discuss these memories with his mother, she revealed that his father had hoped for a robust leader as a son. This helped Amar understand why he had always felt as if he never measured up. Amar's mother further admitted that it was his father's insistence that led to Amar being weaned at just three months old.

With these multiple narrative threads emerging, Amar's story of his adult-onset GERD began to make sense. He realized that a part of him remained stuck in his own childhood, as long as he had unprocessed feelings about a deeply rooted sense of inadequacy. With this newfound understanding, Amar saw his GERD symptoms as a physical manifestation of a recurring theme in his life story. His reinterpretation of his story allowed him to see his GERD as an ally in his desire for approval and a sense of self-worth.

The hermeneutic circle: Whole-of-life

Developing a whole-of-life awareness of your GERD is the pinnacle of your journey where you get to assemble the pieces of your story into its ultimate meaning and you also get to make new choices about who you are. This is the essence of healing, which not only involves the resolution of physical symptoms, but also reconnection of the different parts that make us whole.

If you allow room for the spiritual "I Am" dimension, it is possible to see healing as a form of reconnection with something greater than self. My own subjective perspective is that the universe is one indivisible whole composed entirely of the "fabric" that is Consciousness. Seen in this way, our personal healing manifests as the expansion of Consciousness in which everyone and everything is the beneficiary. However, Consciousness is just one label, and you are always welcome to substitute this for another. The scientists may prefer the term energy, and the religious will have God and its many variants. Whatever label we choose, I believe it is always helpful to experience the underlying unity of formlessness, and not only the superficial separation of forms.

Back to Amar's story:

Today, Amar recognizes that his symptoms were the physical manifestation of a lifelong struggle that really began in his infancy, and which ultimately demanded his attention when unremitting symptoms in early adulthood led to a formal GERD diagnosis. Amar reflected that his adult-onset GERD symptoms coincided with a painful relationship breakup that eventuated in part because he unfairly blamed his partner for unacknowledged feelings around self-worth, as well as his own belief that he could never win his partner's approval.

Amar began to see his GERD as a metaphor for his life, and recognized within this metaphor his need for self-nourishment, self-acceptance and an egoless understanding of self-worth. Through embracing this whole-of-life perspective, Amar found a new way to express an abundant masculinity that did not require external validation from others. Specifically, he associated his whole-of-life challenge and its associated meaning as:

- Gaining acceptance of his masculinity through releasing any concerns around how he perceives others need to see him, whether as a son, a partner, or one day a father himself.

- Choosing to define abundance through an inner awareness of his self-worth, reflecting his own values rather than the top-down values imposed on him as a child and which he continued to demand of himself throughout life until his GERD awakened a need for authenticity.

- Looking for ongoing opportunities for self-nourishment in order to be the best version of himself and therefore able to best serve others.

Identifying any limiting beliefs as they relate to our whole-of-life experience is key to self-healing. Accepting old beliefs (see: *Accepting and reframing feelings*) and choosing new, supportive ones led to Amar healing his GERD. The fact that you are reading his story now is a testament to your own journey and what I maintain can be your own profound healing.

---

1. Christian, H.B., (2015). Subjective dimensions of meaning in the clinical encounter: Unifying personhood and disease. *Energy Psychology: Theory, Research and Treatment,* 7(1): 30–38.

Thirteen

Working with Symbols

Paying attention to symbols of embodied awareness

A symbol is an abstraction that can be used to understand the whole and find meaning. Imagine seeing a motor vehicle or even a horse-drawn cart for the first time. In such circumstances, observing the wheels and their cyclical motion may be critical in *seeing* the vehicle and developing an intuitive understanding of its function. The wheel in this example is a symbol whose observation brings us to the whole. Quite often the whole is not even visible and it is only through direct experience of abstract symbols that we get a sense of its existence. Think of our infinite universe!

GERD is like this when it first announces itself through the appearance of signs and symptoms, which are mere symbols of the whole disease. As we move beyond its superficiality, GERD emerges as a symbol of suffering, and suffering is seen as a symbol of a significant aspect of our lived experience. As we move though its layers, we may see that one person's lived experience with GERD is a symbol of the lived experience of all people living with GERD. Beyond this, we may begin to weave in even deeper layers and view our global humanity as a symbol of our perilous planetary ecosystem; Earth is a symbol of life within the solar system; and our solar system is a symbol of the dynamic movement of our sun and all its heavenly bodies through the Milky Way galaxy, etc.

The point is that when we engage with our GERD, we can only do so by considering the different symbols which the whole of disease encodes.

The human ear—in Traditional Chinese Medicine (TCM)—has for thousands of years been regarded as a *homunculus* in which the whole as well as each part of the body is encoded. In this way it is possible to treat a diseased tissue or organ by targeting its symbolic representation within the ear. US army medics trained in battlefield medicine have used auricular (ear) acupuncture as first aid since 2001. Studies have even documented its effectiveness for use in the emergency department.[1]

Opening to the whole is critical in self-healing. If we think of disease in terms of the disturbed "I Am," then we can understand and heal the disturbance by accessing our underlying story and feelings, and using these as an opportunity to reconnect with the whole. The way we open is limited only by our imagination and the attention we give to self and whatever symbols emerge for us.[2]

"Attention," says psychologist and bestselling author Steve Taylor, "is an alchemy that turns dullness to beauty and anxiety to ease."[3] But this attention need not be limited to our feelings and whatever else lies within us. Our attention also brings its alchemy when we direct it into the environment around us. Henry David Thoreau explains it this way:

> *"What lies before us and what lies behind us are small matters compared to what lies within us. And when we bring what is within out into the world, miracles happen."*

This bringing "what is within" out into the world is the domain of our imagination, which allows us to work with symbols to bridge the inner and outer aspects of where our attention flows. Whereas in the past you would have regarded these aspects as separate, hopefully now you also have a sense of their unity. Thus, we could look inwardly then outwardly, and see something of ourselves in the environment around us. And the reverse is also true.

As an example, a prisoner may sit inside his prison cell and see only the outward evidence of his imprisonment. If he then looked inwards, it is unlikely that he would have any sense of freedom at that moment. Yet, another prisoner might have a profound sense of his own creativity and sees not his confinement but instead the freedom to explore his creativity. He could then expect to find in the products of his creativity—be it music, art, food, even his relationship with self or other—the symbols of his freedom.

Finding symbols for GERD in nature and creativity

We can use the symbols of nature to find meaning. The bear, for example, is a symbol of courage, the butterfly a symbol of transformation, and the dog a symbol of loyalty. Nature's symbols have been interpreted since ancient times and remain a source of connection with the natural world for people who interpret such symbols. We can apply these same symbols to find meaning in our GERD.

Astrology

Astrology uses the dynamic movements and predicted relative positions of the major celestial bodies at the moment and location of a person's birth to help make sense of their personal attributes, and subsequent life events and relationships. The twelve signs of the zodiac are metaphors for the order and complexity of human experience and can be used to simplify our perceptions of ourselves. If astrology appeals to you, it could be used to explore the meaning of your GERD.

Example: Victoria, a Libra, uses her sign's affinity for balance to explore her GERD and begins to recognize how her tendency to prioritize others' needs over her own leads her to crisis points where she has "nothing more to give." At these times her GERD symptoms are at their worst. She realizes that her path to wholeness requires her to prioritize her own needs while continuing to explore the deeper meaning behind her problematic selflessness.

Cultural values and customs

Do you have any practices that are an essential part of your ethnic identity and/or culture? Such customs are a critical part of well-being, but often become threatened or corrupted when another cultural identity dominates. What are the symbols then of your cultural oppression? And what are the symbols of your way back to cultural well-being? Do cultural practices such as healing with native plants, carving, massage, song, prayer, making and playing traditional instruments, weaving, performing arts, and sacred journeys play a possible role in your wholeness?

Example: Moana, a Māori woman coping with GERD, finds comfort in her traditional weaving practice as she creates a traditional flax basket or kete. She reflects on how each strand represents the interconnected threads of her wholeperson, and notices the weakness of the fibers she unconsciously selected to represent her GERD. Rather than discarding the fibers, Moana reflects on her manager's perceptions of her weakness in her role and becomes suddenly angry, yelling out, "I work my guts off for him." Her own father died on the job and she didn't get to know her grandfather because he drowned at sea while providing kai moana for the family. She vowed to reclaim her family's mana by weaving layers of abundance into her kete that would serve as a symbol of hers and her family's resilience.

Financial systems

The Fibonacci sequence, which gives us the golden ratio, is an example of a natural geometry that is applied on a daily basis to our financial systems, including the share and currency trading markets. Although we typically regard such systems through the lenses of chaos, randomness or macroeconomics, manmade markets as for natural systems have an underlying order and symmetry. Within these markets, the price index of any share or currency pair irrepressibly follows the patterns of the golden ratio, reflecting the collective unconscious fear (bear) and greed (bull) cycles of the entire population of investors and traders.

Example: David, a trader, uses his fresh understanding of GERD to reflect on the parallels between the growth and decay of the markets he observes and the deeper layers of his personal ambitions. He realizes that his hunger for success often blinds him to the other domains of his life, which he neglects in favor of prioritizing abundance. He comes to understand that true wealth involves the intangible things he gets to keep, and not money which is simply a medium of exchange through which he transacts his deals.

Five elements

The elements of earth, fire, steel, water and wood are represented in the therapeutic discipline of Five Elements acupuncture. The serpent throughout history represents kundalini energy and forms the caduceus in medicine. Herbs, stones and crystals are used in healing, with their unique energetic signatures symbolic of the diverse energetic resonances of the different aspects of body-mind. The humble rainbow is a symbol of abundance, connection, illusion and light. If any of these creativities resonate with you, I encourage you to further explore them in the context of your GERD.

Example: Ethan, who struggles with GERD and harbors a profound fear of snakes, wonders if there could be a connection between the two. Recognizing that kundalini energy is coiled and dormant, Ethan begins to see his illness as a manifestation of something he is unable to express. He eventually recognizes this as a base level of anxiety that he learned years ago to disconnect from; his family circumstances growing up were "hard to take." He uses his ongoing journaling to symbolically uncoil the serpent's energy—his anxiety—and begins to use this to transform all areas of his life.

Numbers

Have you ever been watching a movie and noticed the attention that film-makers give to numbers and related symbols? Movies are themselves a study in symbolism, with each scene carefully enhanced using a range of symbolic elements that come together "in the can." In the movies, predetermined numbers are often portrayed in vehicle number plates, street signs, and in appointing sets with objects that represent a numeric value. These are not random, but are instead carefully used to represent the movie's themes. Numbers achieve this by appealing to the unconscious mind, which is constantly scanning the environment for patterns and symmetries.

Some people experience the 11:11 phenomenon, which involves repeated observations of the number 11 in combination with itself (i.e., 11:11), its multiples (e.g, 5:55), or the number 9 (e.g., 9/11). Meaning is subjectively determined, but many people take comfort from the seemingly non-random, synchronous occurrence of these numbers and the universal order it represents.

On a personal note, I have observed 9/11 symbology for many years, but only recently learned this was the date that my mother attempted suicide when I was six years old. Before I resolved my hay fever, its symptoms were especially bad around this time of year. Nature's verdant bounty in springtime—as September is marked in the southern hemisphere where I live—is merely a surface aspect of the allergy puzzle.

So have a think about the numbers that could be important in understanding your GERD. What time of year or days of the week are symptoms worse for you and why? Are there other numerical ways that you can relate to your GERD? Why are these important?

Relational mirrors

You assist your journey when you observe the different kinds of mirrors present in your life. By mirrors I do not just mean the reflective glass in your bathroom; our life mirrors are more subtle than that. Any relationship is a potential mirror, whether it is our relationship with nature, another person, or self. When you see an animal in nature that frightens you, what is the true source of your fear? When you look into another's eyes, who do you see if not yourself? When you look at another's artwork, what do you see if not an aspect of your own experience? And when you look in your bathroom mirror, what do you sense from the image staring back at you?

As you learn to identify the value of all your relationships, you begin to dive below the surface and thus become aware of the important information being reflected back at you. The more you learn to listen to your "I Am," the better you become at reaching an answer.

Example: Michelle, living with GERD, begins to understand her condition by observing the various mirrors in her life that awaken her to her own feeling state. While walking in nature, she notices the lizard that she disturbs and feels this disturbance in her stomach. Gazing into her partner's eyes, she realizes that their shared struggles with communication often mirror her own internal conflicts, prompting her to explore the deeper emotional truths that she needs to share. Reflecting on her artwork, which features chaotic patterns, she sees for the first time her need for containment, and the secrets she cannot risk spilling. Finally, looking into her bathroom mirror, she confronts her reflection with curiosity rather than judgment and sees not only her pain, but a strong woman on a path of understanding and healing.

Sacred geometry

Sacred geometry refers to the recurring geometric patterns that are readily observable in nature. Ancient humans not only recognized these patterns, but incorporated nature's designs into their own creativities. Today we can see the same sacred geometric features in architecture, art, corporate logos, machinery, medicine, music, and religious symbolism to name a few applications.

Religion and more recently the military have co-opted the divine goddess, turning her into a symbol of fear, masculine power and war while simultaneously erasing her history. The dangerous and fearsome excesses of the unbalanced masculine principle along with diminishment of the sacred feminine principle provide an explanation for much of the contemporary challenges of humanity.

Whatever our gender, we all have an equal claim to both our masculinity and femininity. For any men who are guffawing in discomfort right now, I recommend *The hidden spirituality of men: Ten metaphors to awaken the sacred masculine* by Matthew Fox.[4] As we saw earlier with James, Maria and Amar, gender-related themes in general are well worth exploring in the context of your GERD and other diseases. Speaking as a man still learning to embrace his feminine side, our reconnection as men with archetypes that embrace a more holistic sense of masculinity that values compassion, creativity and receptivity will not only support social harmony, but provide personal fulfillment too.

Spirit animals and mythological characters

If you had to choose one animal to be your spirit animal and one character to be your mythological character, which ones would you choose? And why? Start journaling with these symbols to see how they might tie into your story.

Tarot

Originally devised as a way of secretly passing on ideas banned by the church, Tarot is—like any symbol—a mirror of a deeper phenomenon. If you have a deck, pull out three cards at random with the intention of using these cards to teach you about your GERD and help uncover its meaning.

Unveiling further creative possibilities

While it is impossible to provide an exhaustive list of symbols, we can say that humanity has been busy since ancient times finding meaning from innumerable sources and interpreting many of them. Practical applications include personal growth and healing, food production and nutrition, clothing and textiles, design and construction, arts and crafts, and love and relationships. From the perspective of disease in general and your GERD specifically, the main emphasis is on being open to meaning found in those potential symbols that most resonate for you.

Adopting a wholeperson, meaning-based story approach to living free of GERD can seem a bit like unwinding an infinite tangle of string. But so too can it seem daunting finding answers to some of the biggest questions we all have as human beings. If you could bring yourself closer to a deep acceptance of the whole of humanity by finding your own answers to some of these questions, you would make the effort would you not? And what if learning to live free of your own disease was a key part of this acceptance? You would have to make the effort then, right?

So if you ever find yourself questioning your motivation to continue, there are plenty of symbolic reminders of humanity's tireless search for meaning. Many Shinto temples have two demon dog statues guarding the entrance, the dogs representing paradox and confusion as the guardians of truth. Many people are fascinated by the lives and realms of royalty, yet never pause to consider that they too are a queen or king, cloaked in a busy life while ruling over an inner kingdom they know little or nothing about. And we have the polarizing symbols of politics, science and religion to remind us that our own ideas of truth may be quite different to another's.

What we do share is this innate desire for meaning, even if we cannot agree on what it is and how to find it. As long as we recognize our individuality, any meaning must be our own to find, which requires us to face our inner turmoil with courage, self-compassion and wisdom. When we are courageous, we can be different to others and know that although our journey is lonely at times, there is merit in being different. When we have compassion for ourselves, we can cope with others' judgments and even find compassion for their situation. And when we are open to our inner wisdom, we are reminded of the importance of engaging our hearts through appreciation, gratitude and creativity.

So how do you choose to express your creativity? Is it through crafts, dance, drawing, film-making, food, gardening, music, painting, poetry, pottery, sculpture, sports, or another creative medium? Do you find freedom in color, dimensionality, light, motif, mood, movement, or perspective? What does working or playing or creating in a free and unrestricted manner look like? In the words of C.G. Jung:

> *"Your vision will become clear only when you can look into your own heart. Who looks outside, dreams; who looks inside, awakes."*

If you're still stuck, here are a couple of further suggestions:

- Light a candle with the intention of parting the veil of your protective psyche or burning your favorite incense for a shift in mood.

- Thinking of your favorite vehicle, write down your thoughts about which part of it represents your GERD and why. Do it stream-of-consciousness style so you do not have a chance to filter your thoughts. Write for at least five minutes and go big on the details.

- Take the following symbols and write a short story of your GERD, stream-of-consciousness style. Work for five minutes writing down your ideas for the following: Temple, rooster, egg, ball, snake, pig.

Exercise 13.1: Dream journaling for GERD symbolism

Illnesses such as GERD often appear symbolically in dreams, making our dreams worth considering to connect unconscious material directly to our symptoms. Dream work can illuminate fresh perspectives, offering insights into both the psychological as well as somatic aspects of illness. A word of caution: Many books have been written on the subject of dream interpretation, and can be enormously helpful. But you are the only qualified interpreter of your own dreams.

Dream journaling is a great way to channel your unconscious and unlock the meaning it holds. When you are working with dreams, it is a bit like exercising a muscle: If you have not used it in a while it can be a bit painful at first, but regular attention will make harvesting its treasures easier and more rewarding over time.

Here are a few tips for journaling about your dreams to find meaning from your GERD:

Start by setting your intention to catch your dreams

By telling yourself before you go to sleep or upon waking from a dream that "I'll remember this one," you are using the power of your intention to leverage the value of your dreams. You can even be a bit more specific in your intention, as in "The next dream I remember will teach me something valuable about my GERD."

When you wake from your dream

Upon waking after a dream, grab your journal right away and make notes to clarify the dream you have just had. Write about the dream's setting and events along with any feelings that came up.

Focus on your subjective experience

At this initial stage of journaling about your dream, do not think about what it means, but instead focus on the subjective experience of being inside your dream. Describe the experience itself.

Connect your dream to your life

Once you have captured, clarified and described your dream from your inside perspective, now is the time to connect your dream to your life. This is where the meaning happens and it may arrive like an "aha" moment. Try not to force this, but rather let it happen of its own accord.

Respond to your dream

When you have the meaning, it is time to respond to your dream. Start by asking yourself what you are going to do with this meaning, what greater good it serves, and how it might change things for you. Write this down in your journal because these and other ideas will be useful when we get to the final section of this book on *Working with feelings*.

Exercise 13.2: Discovering nature's symbols in your story

Here's an exercise to help you turn your chosen symbol into meaning for your GERD. By engaging deeply with nature's symbols, you may uncover new layers to your story and your relationship with GERD. Enjoy this reflective journey!

1. **Reflect on your symbol:** Take a moment to reflect on the symbols in nature that you most resonate with. Make a

note of at least three different symbols that hold significance in your life.

2. **Explore these symbols for possible meaning:** For each symbol, note down why you find it meaningful. Consider what—or who—it reminds you of; does it evoke a specific person, event or place?

3. **Connect to your GERD story:** Imagine using these symbols to narrate your experience with GERD. How might these symbols change, enrich or even embellish your story? Note down your ideas and possible connections.

4. **Journal your thoughts:** Record your reflections in your journal, capturing any feelings as well as insights as you continue to explore the meaning behind each symbol.

5. **Expand your set of symbols:** Choose three additional symbols from nature that you haven't previously considered. Think of novel and imaginative ways to weave these new symbols into your GERD story.

6. **Notice any physical sensations:** As you engage with all these symbols and journal your reflections, pay close attention to any sensations in your body. Do you feel tension, are you holding your breath, what other sensations are you experiencing and where in your body do you notice them?

7. **Document these physical sensations:** Journal your observations of these physical sensations. If you could name them, what names would you give to each and why?

Exercise 13.3: Recreating your GERD experience

An alternative to the above exercise is to recreate your GERD or some aspect of it using a creative medium of your choice. This does not need to be a finished piece, so when you have a working model or abstraction of your GERD, look within the symbol you have created for the presence of other symbols, much like you were opening a Russian doll.

1. **Choose your creative medium:** Select a creative medium that most resonates with you, such as drawing, painting, sculpture, vlogging, or any other form of creative expression that appeals to you.

2. **Use this medium to recreate your GERD:** While recreating your GERD or an aspect of it, focus on crafting your working model with the aim being to express your experience.

3. **Explore the symbols within:** Once you have created your representation, take a moment to look within your creation for other symbols, considering new layers of meaning, previously hidden elements, or nuances that may reveal themselves as you simply observe your creation with your full attention.

4. **Reflect in your journal:** Journal your thoughts about how these secondary symbols change, enrich, embellish, or add depth to the narrative of your GERD experience.

5. **Seek fresh perspectives:** After finishing your initial reflections, return to your creation. This time, shift your perspective: Soften your gaze, hum, blink, or scratch an imaginary itch. Engage all your senses and approach the piece with a fresh mindset.

6. **Notice any surprises:** As you take this new perspective, note down any surprising observations, feelings or fresh symbols that emerge from your creation.

7. **Inventive integration:** Consider imaginative ways to incorporate these fresh symbols into your GERD story. How might they impact the narrative you wish to convey?

8. **Tune into your body:** Throughout this exploration, maintain an acute awareness of your body. Notice any physical sensations, shifts in energy, or emotional responses that arise during this process.

9. **Document your insights:** Finally, journal any additional thoughts or insights, reflecting on how this exercise has reshaped your understanding of your GERD experience.

---

1. Jan, A.L., Aldridge, E.S., Rogers, I.R., Visser, E.J., Bulsara, M.K., & Niemtzow, R.C., (2017). Does ear acupuncture have a role for pain relief in the emergency setting? A systematic review and meta-analysis. *Medical Acupuncture,* 29(5): 276-289.

2. Feinstein, D., & Krippner, S., (2008). Personal mythology: Using ritual, dreams, and imagination to discover your inner story. Santa Rosa, CA, USA; Energy Psychology Press/Elite Books.

3. Taylor, S., (2015). The calm center: Reflections and meditations for spiritual awakening. Novato, CA, USA; New World Library.

4. Fox, M., (2008). The hidden spirituality of men: Ten metaphors to awaken the sacred masculine. Novato, CA, USA; New World Library.

Fourteen

Charting Your Symptoms

Begin with a symptom list

Making a chart of your symptoms can provide a powerful visual depiction of the connections that exist between your disease and the events in your life. This approach brings your GERD into the now and allows you to see in real-time how your experiences are reflected dynamically in your body.

When you develop and maintain your chart, you are not only recording any symptom fluctuations. You are also mapping your mood and stress levels, and learning to associate these with whatever else is going on in your life.

Start by making a list of specific symptoms in order of their importance or severity to you. If it helps, choose your symptoms from the following list. In addition to this list, you may have other symptoms which are not typically considered to be GERD-related, but which nevertheless cause you regular discomfort. Feel welcome to add them to your own list. GERD symptoms vary widely among individuals.

1. **Heartburn:** A classic symptom of GERD characterized by a burning sensation in the chest, often rising toward the throat; typically occurs after eating or when lying down.

2. **Regurgitation:** A classic symptom of GERD characterized by the sensation of acid backing up into the throat or mouth; often accompanied by a sour or bitter taste.

3. **Dysphagia:** Difficulty with swallowing, which can also be associated with pain (odynophagia).

4. **Chest pain:** Discomfort or pain in the chest that may feel sharp, burning, or pressure-like; can mimic heart-related issues.

5. **Chronic cough:** A persistent cough that can range from mild to severe, and which is often worse after meals or during the night.

6. **Sore throat:** A persistent or recurrent hoarseness or sore throat, which can be mistaken for a cold or allergies.

7. **Laryngitis:** Inflammation of the larynx, which causes hoarseness or loss of voice due to acid exposure.

8. **Bad breath (halitosis):** An unpleasant odor emitted from the mouth.

9. **Asthma:** New-onset or worsening symptoms involving wheezing and/or shortness of breath.

10. **Globus sensation:** The feeling of a lump or a sensation of fullness in the throat or chest.

11. **Nausea:** A feeling of discomfort in the stomach, which can be accompanied by an urge to vomit especially for severe reflux episodes.

12. **Dyspepsia:** Indigestion is often experienced as discomfort or pain in the upper abdomen, most commonly after eating or drinking.

13. **Bloating and gas:** Other symptoms associated with GERD include belching, bloating and gas.

Creating your chart

Now that you have a list of symptoms ranked in terms of how much suffering they cause you, choose one high on your list that tends to have a clear onset and offset, or which comes in bouts or attacks. Alternatively, if any of your symptoms worsen and improve synchronously, consider grouping them as a single symptom cluster. Having selected an ideal candidate, it is time to explore your symptom(s) through the use of a chart.

The example chart below illustrates Jamal's classic symptoms of heartburn and regurgitation severity—which he grouped together as a single symptom cluster in bold ink—and his mood, which he overlaid in light ink. The mood scale represents general mood rather than how a person feels about their symptoms. Both symptom severity and mood are charted over time, with three data points for morning (am), midday (mid) and evening (pm) for each of the seven days of the chart. There is also a space at the bottom of each day for short comments relating to key events or experiences. You can download a template chart to record your own daily and weekly GERD symptoms and general mood. See the link at the end of the chapter for details.

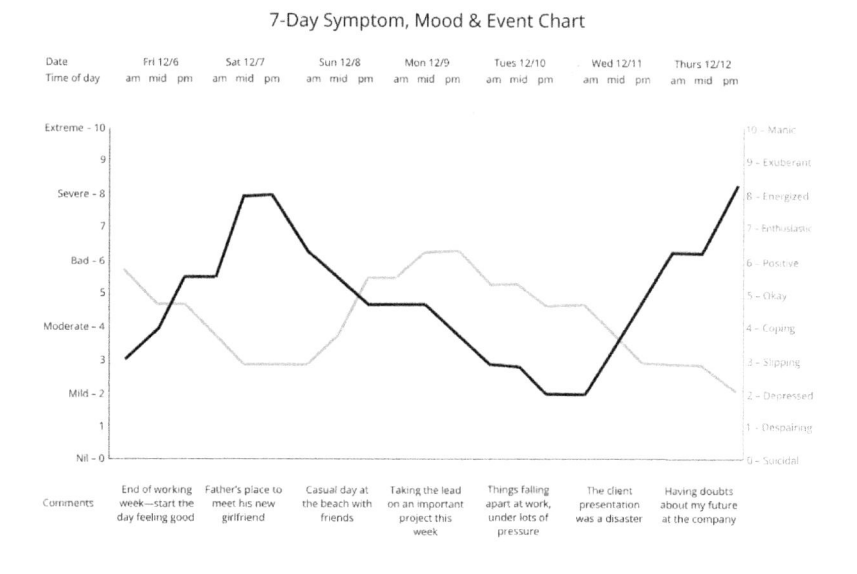

Figure 14.1: *Jamal's symptom-mood chart showing changes in symptom severity of heartburn/regurgitation and mood over time.*

When creating your own chart, use the vertical symptom scale to rate your chosen symptom(s) on a 0–10 scale where 10 represents extreme severity and 0 means the symptom is not present at all.

Next, use the vertical mood scale to rate your subjective mood, also on a 0–10 scale. If none of the words for mood used in the example chart resonates with you, think instead of words like up or down, relaxed or tense, or calm or anxious.

Be sure to record your actual mood rather than what you want your mood to be. At any moment in time, we are all somewhere on this mood scale. Most people experience continuous fluctuations between "energized," represented by a mood score of 8, and "slipping," represented by a mood score of 3; 10 represents extreme mania and 0 is suicidal.

> **IMPORTANT: If you score yourself a 0 or 10 at any time for your mood, I strongly urge you to seek medical help. The world needs you in it. You are valued and loved, even if this does not seem to be your reality right now.**

Interpreting symptom-mood charts

In Jamal's chart, there is a strong and clear relationship between the severity of his heartburn and regurgitation symptoms and his general mood scored at the same time intervals three times daily over the week.

Jamal showed worsening symptoms and a corresponding drop in mood around the time he visited his father and his father's new girlfriend. His symptoms and mood both improved when, the following day, he relaxed with his friends at the beach. His work week started well when he was given the lead on an important project, but when things started to spiral out of control and an important client presentation ended in disaster, his symptoms escalated. At the same time, Jamal's mood declined into depression as he began to have doubts over his future.

Jamal's experiences highlight the strong connections between unexplored emotional states and the physical symptoms of GERD, such as heartburn and regurgitation. The visit to his father and introduction to his father's new girlfriend seemed to evoke complex feelings for Jamal, perhaps involving unresolved family dynamics. Jamal needs to focus on these embodied feelings and any associated thoughts in order to uncover a possible somatic metaphor, which is the entry point into a deeper understanding of his story. What we do know is that Jamal's bodymind is having difficulty processing these layered feelings.

Jamal's subsequent improvement in both his symptoms and mood after spending time with friends suggests a protective element (see: *The five P's*) associated with the nurturing aspect of social bonds. It's also likely that Jamal regards the beach environment as a safe space to unwind and rejuvenate. Whenever we identify our happy places, it is always useful to reflect on what are the accompanying feelings and thoughts. As much as I am *not* a fan of the cognitive-behavioral therapeutic (CBT) model (see: *Getting therapeutic support for GERD*), it nevertheless can have positive applications in our healing. In this case, if Jamal were to recognize the positive thoughts associated with going to the beach, he could use the same thoughts to reframe a negative experience, such as going to see his father/father's new girlfriend. Provided Jamal is able to identify and adequately process his underlying feelings (which CBT does not enable us to do), then having positive reframes for experiences that we ordinarily find stressful is useful.

Jamal's initial excitement about leading an important work project aligns with the boost in his mood. The combination of positive expectation and self-agency typically enhances well-being. However, a positive expectation can be a two-edged sword as it proved to be in Jamal's case when challenges arose and his important presentation did not go well leading to disappointment and overwhelm. Jamal clearly struggled to cope with this work pressure and the perceived failure he had around his own performance. The resulting fears and doubts about his future only continued to fuel his worsening symptoms, as his mood slipped further into depression.

Based on what we do know about Jamal, including the location and nature of his symptoms, my encouragement for him would be to consider any related somatic metaphors. Examples that may fit with his symptoms *and* story include a hunger for love (stomach and heart) and expecting too much (stomach and mouth), as well as metaphors around feeling let down, disappointment, and self-worth (see: *The stomach as metaphor*).

Take a close look at the chart and confirm for yourself how Jamal's worsening symptoms coincided with a drop in his mood. Your own chart may or may not show a trend as clear as Jamal's. Either way, keep monitoring your own symptom and mood fluctuations for a few weeks to look for patterns.

Also try charting other symptoms—either together as for Jamal's synchronous experience of heartburn with regurgitation—or individually, which works better when your symptoms appear separately to one another. You could chart individual symptoms together, but use different colors to represent the different symptoms. Remember to include your general mood changes. Assigning a score for your symptoms and mood at regular intervals is a subjective exercise. But remember, you are the expert.

Mood awareness

If your mood chart shows a straight line in the exuberant, energized or enthusiastic bands, you are either a rare individual indeed *or* you are not in touch with your feelings (see: *We are trained not to feel*). People intrinsically understand that it is normal to experience a fluctuation in mood. From a young age, we are exposed to a wide range of emotional experiences and we begin to appreciate that feelings can change based on various external events and relational interactions. As we mature, we begin to make the connection between our thoughts as amplifiers of our feelings, and so we develop an internal sense of rhythm in our mood as a result. We are also adept at anticipating changes in mood based on past experiences, which fosters coping strategies and enables us to navigate challenging times with the understanding that our emotional state will improve.

If you have a relatively flat line for your mood, you are actually *more* likely to experience physical symptoms.[1] This is because your bodymind responds to any detachment from significant feelings by placing these issues into bodily form. This is how the bodymind gets our attention!

It is not uncommon for people to experience life along a narrow okay/coping band. If this is you, it is likely that you do not have much to get excited about. With the exception of your GERD and any other conditions, you may believe that you do not have much to complain about. People with this flat affect may be more down than they realize, but use their defenses to keep depression at bay.

Finally, some people will not see a correlation between their symptoms and mood. Yet, when they make a connection between their symptoms and story, their symptoms improve anyway. This chart will not be useful for everyone since charting relies on measuring something that is experienced subjectively. The major focus of this exercise is to increase your awareness of the relationship between story and symptoms.

Your Home Remedy for Acid Reflux Disease

Free Companion Resources

Enhance your journey with *Your Home Remedy for Acid Reflux Disease: Live, Eat and Heal Abundantly* by unlocking a treasure trove of FREE Companion Resources. Dive into symptom-mood charts, exclusive audio exercises, and a transformative MindBody workbook designed to accelerate your healing from acid reflux disease/GERD. And this is just the beginning—stay tuned for more bonus content coming your way!

Don't wait—visit the link below to gain instant access and enhance your journey to wellness today!

HOWARDCHRISTIAN.COM/READER-COMPANION-RESOURCES

Live, Eat and Heal Abundantly

---

1. Broom, B., (1997). Somatic illness and the patient's other story. London, UK; Free Association Books.

Part III: Working with Feelings

*"It is not selfish or narcissistic to love yourself.
It is your first and foremost responsibility."*

— Alan Cohen

Fifteen

Affect, Emotion, Feeling and Communication

Affective behavior in infancy

We each have the potential to experience and describe an enormous array of feelings. Joy, astonishment, overwhelm, worthlessness, betrayal, embarrassment and abandonment are just a few examples of the spectrum of feelings we have collectively put a name to. As storytellers, regaling our life's stories would be pointless if not for the feelings that our experiences evoke. Feelings are the symbols that make our stories relatable, memorable and meaningful. But to become the symbolic devices of our stories, our feelings first have to undergo a journey of their own. And it is a journey that begins in infancy.

If we look at infants, we can observe seven basic facial expressions that alert us to what the infant is experiencing in response to an external stimulus. One, with baby's eyebrows up and eyes blinking, baby expresses surprise or startle. Two, further exposure to the same stimulus may evoke interest or excitement, with baby's eyebrows down, eyes tracking, and with an attitude of looking and listening. Three, baby may arch their eyebrows, the corners of the mouth will turn down, tears may appear, and a rhythmic sobbing begins—baby is letting us know that they are distressed or anguished. Four, for a baby to show us contempt or disgust, they will sneer with the upper lip raised. Five, baby's frown, clenched jaw and red face are the features of baby's anger or rage. Six, with baby's eyes frozen open, face pale and sweaty, and body trembling with their hair erect, baby shows their fear or terror. Seven, soothed and safe, baby's smile returns, lips are wide and outward, and their breathing is slow and deep, signaling baby's contentment or joy.

This *affective behavior* is what we see on the outside, but there is a lot more going on inside than just the actions of the facial muscles. What we observe in our own and others' affective behavior reflects the body's generalized physiologic responses. These include breathing, heart rate, dilation of the pupils, respiration rate, body temperature, sweating, gastrointestinal motility, etc. They also include the accompanying physical bodily sensations, which we can think of as *emotions*.

Affective behavior as communication

By attuning to our emotions, we can begin to articulate the accompanying subjective state with the help of symbols (e.g., preverbal, verbal and nonverbal language). In this way, affects undergo transformation as we attune to the corresponding emotions. With further differentiation, cognition and articulation, emotions become feelings.

Affective behavior is useful for infants because it alerts their caregiver to some unmet need. We can therefore think of affect as a primitive form of communication, which gets increasingly more complex as a baby grows and learns and relates to others. The key point here is that babies—and adults too—use affective behavior to communicate a need.

Upon recognizing the baby's message, the responsive caregiver will fulfill the need in the form of comfort, warmth, food, love and connection. This care gives the baby an internal sense of security and resilience that comes from having their bodily affects regulated. Critically, this care also teaches the developing baby how to regulate their own bodily affects and, later, their emotions and feelings.

But the baby's message is lost if their caregiver cannot attune to their affective behavior. With the affect unrecognized and the baby's accompanying need unmet, affect regulation is unable to occur. If this is a constant theme in the baby's life, they will not develop an internal sense of security and safety.

Instead, their physiology is unstable, their breathing is shallow and irregular, their heart rhythm lacks the variability of a healthy child, they respond disproportionately to perceived threats, and their learning is adversely impacted. The baby struggles to self-soothe and looks outside of themselves for ways to fulfill their needs. As the child grows, they bring their difficulties into their relationships. And this begins a vicious, unconscious cycle of relational dysfunction (see: *Feelings as connection*).

Attuning to—and naming—our feelings requires a conscious choice

Fortunately, we can learn at any point in our life journey to consciously regulate our embodied emotional state. We can do this with some targeted activities that help us attune to and process the negative aspects of our stories. We can also awaken from a dominant negative feeling state to a dominant positive one through the power of intention, and the use of targeted techniques such as those described in *Accepting and reframing feelings through energy psychology*. We can also use our positive feeling states to show care for others, which helps them shift to a positive feeling state too.

The reality is that no matter how bleak our past,[1] we all have the capacity to transform our embodied emotions into subjective feeling qualities that we can give a name to. By naming our feelings, they lose their charge and we can begin to accept and even reframe them. This helps us to move beyond suffering and to heal any underlying disease.

But to name and work with our feelings, we must first attune to them. And before we can attune to these feelings, we might need to recognize and overcome the subliminal training we received as young children; subliminal training that defends us from having to experience our authentic feelings.

Anger, fear, grief and shame are not intangible, irrational concepts that come into being only in the space between our ears, serving little purpose other than to make us feel bad. Rather, we know them as feelings because we have first *felt* them in our bodies as emotions. We give them a name so that we can express them through language.

Nor do these feelings simply vanish because we intellectually understand them. Yes, cognition is important when seeking ways to release our stuck feelings. But charged emotions such as those we develop in response to trauma must be directly addressed at the body level. So if you no longer want to "burn" with anger, or "shake" in fear, or "choke" with grief or "hide" in shame, it is time to do something different from what you have normally done to this point.

Exercise 15.1: Conscious breath work

It may surprise you to learn that we are biologically programmed to experience and release emotions *physically*. Again, we can look to infants to see the truth of this statement. Infants instinctively express their pleasurable *and* painful emotions through leg kicking, arm waving, back arching, head waggling, and everyone's favorite, erupting in piercing screams.

Breathing, while also an instinctive process, is something that most people today do not do well. We are a society of "bad-breathers" because we are stuck in fear. An instinctive response to fear is to hold your breath, but in case you haven't noticed, modern societies thrive on dishing out a cold diet of fear. The result is that we get locked into a vicious cycle of shallow breathing that not only entrains the diaphragm to work against its natural rhythm, but also creates a fear-readiness state.

Again, we can look to infants for instruction on how to breathe correctly. When an infant breathes in, notice how their belly expands outward. And when they breathe out, their belly contracts inward toward their spine. Their breathing is slow, deep, full and regular, and normally achieved through nostril breathing. This healthy breathing cycle removes carbon dioxide from the body and increases available oxygen and energy.

It also promotes the release of deep-seated emotions.

This simple breath exercise uses your conscious awareness to bring you back to a health-giving breath cycle.

1. Sit comfortably with your eyes closed.

2. Begin by simply noticing your breathing.

3. Now, take a deep breath in through the nose, allowing your belly to gently expand outward, gradually filling your lungs and finally your chest.

4. Breathe slowly out through the nose, noticing your belly contracting toward your spine, using your diaphragm to push the last of your breath out of your lungs.

5. Return to simply noticing your breathing, paying attention to the pause between each breath, the depth of your breath, and its slow, rhythmic cycle.

Repeat this exercise for 2–3 minutes each day until your natural breathing rhythm is re-established and you are breathing like a baby once more! Notice your increased energy levels and the heightened sense of peace.

---

1. Levy, T.M., & Orlans, M., (2014). Corrective attachment therapy: Methods and interventions. In T.M. Levy, & M. Orlans (Eds.), Attachment, trauma, and healing: Understanding and treating attachment disorder in children, families, and adults (pp. 186-233). London, UK: Jessica Kingsley Publishers.

Sixteen

We Are Trained Not To Feel

We are trained from a young age not to feel. There are many ways this occurs, and we will discuss seven of them. All happen at an unconscious level, so neither the trainer nor the trainee is aware of the impact on our feelings.

This being trained not to feel starts in relationship with the significant people in our lives, including parents, caregivers, siblings, teachers, coaches, religious leaders, and our peers. These significant people are invariably unaware of their own unconscious messaging so this chapter is not about finding fault.

This learning happens when we are young, and therefore sponges for new information. To our further detriment, this unconscious messaging is reinforced in the media, the entertainment industry, the classroom, the law courts, the military, health clinics and hospital rooms, boardrooms, in fact in every segment of society.

Following are seven ways we are trained not to feel along with seven ways that we can be more conscious parents or caregivers, or even just caring folk who desire a more feeling world in which everyone thrives.

Distraction

Common scenario

As you go about the daily busy-ness of toddlerhood, you fall down and scrape your knee. You are hurt, there is no doubt. You scream your distress and your caregiver, who is nearby, immediately comes to your aid. Fearing judgment or a backlash from passersby, your caregiver distracts you from your physical pain and emotional anguish by shushing and handing you a toy.

You are encouraged to divert all your attention away from what is going on in your body in favor of your caregiver's own needs, which the toy symbolizes. The pain continues, but because your engagement with the toy pleases your caregiver and those around you, the pain is secondary and therefore relegated in its importance.

Conscious parenting

Children need to learn that their distress is a natural response to a stressor, such as being physically hurt or having a sibling take a toy off them. Rather than distracting a child from their pain, parents and caregivers must show the child that their pain is an important experience for them in that moment. By encouraging the child to *feel* their hurt, we teach them to engage with whatever is present for them in the here and now, giving it their full attention. In this way, they will become champions of their own feelings and they will also learn to recognize hurt in others. Using this empathy, they will become a great source of support for others in times of hurt.

Think of the nuance here as the difference between placing your palm gently on the back of someone who is crying, and rubbing or patting that person's back or shoulder. Done in an intentional way, the former is holding a space for the person, helping them to be present and attune to their distress. The latter gives a different message, perhaps one that they should stop crying now.

Suppression

Common scenario

As a young child, you show your anger when your caregiver violates an interpersonal boundary. This might occur, for example, when the caregiver's action or inaction appears to favor a sibling or causes you loss. Rather than acknowledging your anger, your caregiver instead gets angry with you. They are bigger and more forceful, and your natural response is to feel afraid. Rather than risk showing your anger again, you learn instead that the safe option is to suppress your anger. You do not know it at the time, but this unconscious suppression initiates a lifelong pattern of withholding your anger and having it expressed another way, such as through body illness or behavior.

Conscious parenting

As responsible adults, parents and caregivers need to help young children find ways to deal appropriately with their strong feelings, including anger, fear, grief and shame. This always starts with acknowledging whatever has come up for the child, and requires the caregiver to place the child's needs ahead of their own. By encouraging children in this way, they learn that their strong feelings are natural and important. When their feelings are honored, children also learn the important lesson of self-management.

This does not mean that the caregiver should take an unbounded approach to children's feelings. On the contrary, caregivers need to give the child clear expectations about what is an appropriate expression of anger versus an inappropriate expression of rage. But unless the child's behavior is endangering themselves or others, this moderation will need to occur once the child has had a chance to express and explore their feelings in the moment.

A suitable statement to the over-angry or tantrum-throwing child might be, "I can see you are angry, but you need to calm down." This acknowledges what the child is feeling and gives them a clear expectation of what is required.

Comfort

Common scenario

Giving comfort is a natural and humane response to a child's distress. But dealt with in the wrong way, it can also lead to a lifetime of using comfort to avoid the discomfort of our significant feelings. Imagine a scenario where, as a child, your favorite grandparent died. Rather than encouraging you to be with your feelings of grief, your caregiver instead offered you the comfort of food or video games. Or they left you alone in your grief, and now feeling disconnection as well as grief, you need to find your own source of comfort.

It is not uncommon in times of grief, for example, for people to pull out their hair or pick at their skin. You can imagine how this might become a source of ongoing comfort to someone who, as a child, had been left to work through significant feelings on their own. Alcohol, drugs, exercise, gambling, hoarding, overeating, overworking, sex, screen time, shopping, and impulse control disorders such as dermatillomania and trichotillomania are common sources of comfort in materialistic societies that place the need for comfort ahead of the discomfort of important feelings.

Conscious parenting

When a child needs comfort, it is seldom the right thing to leave them alone. And it is never okay to replace their need for comfort with a comfortable substitute such as food or video games. In times of loss, a child more than ever needs to feel connection. The substitute may well provide short-term comfort, but the trade-off is long-term pain since it will never make up for the break in connection that created the need for emotional closeness in the first place.

On the other hand, having a parent or caregiver who is present for the child during their need for closeness teaches the child that they will be supported in times of loss. In relationship, the child learns that their strong feelings will be validated and that real comfort arrives from a shared experience in which empathy is the glue that binds relationships, families and communities together.

Dissociation

Common scenario

Do you ever feel like you zone out, that things around you begin to look strange or unfamiliar, that you are listening but someone's words do not reach you, or that you simply feel unreal? This dissociation is not uncommon and occurs as either depersonalization—a feeling of separation between yourself and your body—or derealization—a feeling of separation between yourself, other people and objects in your environment. If you do experience dissociation, you may have learned this coping strategy or defense as a response to childhood trauma.

Imagine a scenario in which you were overwhelmed by stressors in your childhood home, or you expressed significant feelings that were dealt with by a caregiver who then shook you, slapped you, or in some other way violated an interpersonal boundary. Your response as a child was to connect to your fight, flight or freeze response, which are instinctual reactions designed to promote survival in the face of danger. When traumatic experiences are recurrent, and initial fight or flight reactions are ineffective, a child's reaction to trauma can evolve into maladaptive coping mechanisms, including disconnecting from the present moment, their feelings and aspects of self to cope with the overwhelming distress. Over time, the child may begin to perceive non-threatening situations as potential sources of trauma, triggering heightened feelings of anxiety and leading the child to dissociate even in safe environments.

This emotional numbing or detachment provides the child with protection from their significant feelings, which ultimately leads to difficulties in forming healthy relationships, ongoing issues with emotional processing, and deeper psychological problems, including anxiety disorders, depression, and post-traumatic stress disorder (PTSD).

Conscious parenting

It is never okay to hit, slap, smack or use any other violent, aggressive or sexual force against a child. Nor is it okay to bombard a child with insults or engage in other forms of bullying behavior in which the intention, however unconscious, is to demean and diminish the child.

> **IMPORTANT:** If you use or think about using any of these behaviors against a child or anyone else, I urge you to seek help immediately. Abusive behavior in any form is never okay. Help is available and it is your responsibility to seek that help.

In addition to feeling connected, children need to develop an appreciation of their own developing autonomy. As such, inviolable rights that we expect as adults must also be extended to children. This ensures that children can feel safe, with the accompanying certainty that they can depend on the significant adults in their lives to look after them.

Since dissociation may also occur in response to natural events such as earthquakes, it is important to reassure children of their safety whenever possible and meaningful to do so. We also need to acknowledge that there are natural phenomena outside our control, but that as adults we are taking steps to lessen any risk to their person.

Denial

Common scenario

Children are frequently denied access to their own feelings growing up. By the time they are adults, many have learned to deny their significant feelings. Examples include when a child is told that their pain is not so bad, their sadness is not so useful, or when someone laughs at their expression of self-worth. These experiences not only diminish the child, but they also reduce the child's ability to feel what is going on within their bodies.

Denial also occurs when a parent or caregiver does something that transgresses a child's boundaries, but rather than acknowledge the impact on the child, they choose instead to justify their actions or deny the child's version of what happened. A form of denial occurs when a parent smother's their child at the first sign of them having an emotional response. If we look at the parent's own motives for their behavior in this situation, it likely stems from an unconscious need to mitigate their own discomfort, or even to place themselves unnecessarily at the center of their child's world.

Denial has an insidious presence in society whereupon individuals and organizations alike refuse to be accountable for their actions, breaching trust and the social capital that is needed to maintain healthy communities.

Conscious parenting

Hopefully, it will now be evident that children need support if they are to safely explore their feelings. They also need to have people in their lives who can validate their feelings. There are few statements with as much power as, "I can see you're angry, and I'd feel angry too if that happened to me."

If you feel the power in that statement, then consider this as a follow-up question: "Whereabouts in your body do you feel angry? Maybe you could point it out to me so I can better understand your anger." Then you could ask them, "What do you need from me so I can help you let go of your anger?" If the child is not yet talking, you could ask them instead, "Would it be okay if I gave you a hug to help you let go of your anger?"

Manipulation

Common scenario

Depending on the dynamics at home, a child may be encouraged to turn their feelings into something other than what they really feel. "If you give me that Big Girl smile, I'll forget how angry you made me and perhaps we'll get an ice cream later on." There are three things that are manipulative about this statement: First, the caregiver asks the child to feel something that they do not feel; second, the caregiver refuses to take responsibility for their own feelings, and instead requires the child to take responsibility; and third, the caregiver uses a bribe to reinforce the value of taking their preferred path.

This transactionalism between parent and child harbors the same interdependency, significance and reciprocity of a transaction between two consenting adults who presumably are each aware of the potential impact of the transaction on their relationship and related outcomes. Only here, there is a significant power differential between the adult and child. Taking this example to a possible outcome, the girl may become a young woman who believes that sex is a duty of her relationship, having first obliged her partner with a smile.

Consider another scenario: "I'll not have you acting like a moody prince in my house. You wipe that pout off your face this minute or I'll..." In this scenario, the child is manipulated into feeling something other than what they feel in order to avoid a potentially painful consequence. Similar to the transactionalism of the previous example, there are consequences to the boy as he grows into a man. He may internalize rather than express his true feelings, or he might replicate these dynamics and become the manipulating and aggressive force of authority in his future relationships. Whichever route he follows, he will experience difficulties coping with conflict and finding the vulnerability required for real intimacy.

Conscious parenting

Manipulation is a dangerous game. Our societies are full of people who, as children, learned to turn their real feelings into something else and who escaped the value of those real feelings in favor of avoiding a penalty or gaining an advantage. In turn, they learn to manipulate the feelings of others.

Compared with the general population, a disproportionately high percentage of CEOs, bureaucrats, clergy, entertainers, journalists, lawyers, media personalities, police officers, politicians, surgeons and people convicted of crimes display a talent for manipulation either because their survival as children depended on it, or their parents sought their children's personal advancement at the expense of their integrity and authenticity.[1] As a society, we all pay the price.

Asking "Why?"

Common scenario

The most insidious way we are taught not to feel may seem harmless enough. When a child feels sad, bad or mad and we ask them, "Why?" we are usually doing so from a place of caring. The fact that we can recognize their distress and want to support them is a good thing because it shows empathy. But in the moment of asking "Why?" we are also guilty of taking the child out of their body and into their thoughts instead.

We are giving priority not to *what* the child is feeling, but the *reason* for this feeling. This necessarily involves cognitive effort that is typically beyond the child's immediate grasp and results in the child making up an answer that has little or nothing to do with the feeling that they have. Then, as adults, we argue, complain, gossip, mismanage, swear, and generally express our negativity, but fail to observe the feelings that give rise to these patterns of behavior.

Conscious parenting

Instead of asking a child, "Why?" when they are hurt or sad, it is enough for us to be with them. Our silence gives them consent to feel. When accompanied by our intentional care, our silence also allows them to feel held and deeply heard (see: *Feelings as connection*). There will come a moment when the sound of your voice is reassuring, but this is not yet the time to ask, "Why?"

Instead, your encouragement will tell them it is okay to feel their hurt. This could be anger, betrayal, bewilderment, anger, pain, whatever. At this time it does not need a name because, to the child, they are simply experiencing their embodied emotions. When the child is ready, they will give this emotion a name—as they have heard you do—and sometimes this is enough. Sometimes the child will need time alone to explore their story. When ready, your child will come back to you. But given the space to feel and your intentional care, your child will know that they are not alone. This is true power.

Exercise 16.1: Emotional awareness questionnaire

Distraction, suppression, comfort, dissociation, denial, manipulation and asking "Why?"—the major strategies we use to defend against our own and others' feelings—occur without our conscious involvement. Even with our consciousness raised and our defenses down, many of us would still struggle to identify important feelings.

The reason for this is that against our backgrounds of learning not to feel, there are common patterns of belief and behavior that we acquire from those around us, which prevent the free flow of authentic feeling. Understanding why our particular circumstances make it hard to identify important feelings helps us to reconnect with those feelings.

One way to this understanding is to acknowledge some common patterns of belief and behavior that you have grown up around and which may persist for you beyond childhood. The following questionnaire is designed to help you reflect on your emotional experiences and patterns from childhood and how they might influence your current emotional self-awareness and expression. For each statement, indicate how much you agree or disagree using the indicated scale.

1. During my childhood, I was not encouraged to express or share my feelings.
   [ ] Strongly disagree
   [ ] Disagree
   [ ] Neutral
   [ ] Agree
   [ ] Strongly agree

2. I see problems in others more easily than I recognize problems in myself.
   [ ] Strongly disagree
   [ ] Disagree

[ ] Neutral
[ ] Agree
[ ] Strongly agree

3. My parents and family members were unwilling to express their own feelings.
   [ ] Strongly disagree
   [ ] Disagree
   [ ] Neutral
   [ ] Agree
   [ ] Strongly agree

4. I believe that I am more naturally in control of my feelings than others.
   [ ] Strongly disagree
   [ ] Disagree
   [ ] Neutral
   [ ] Agree
   [ ] Strongly agree

5. During my childhood, others received my feelings badly.
   [ ] Strongly disagree
   [ ] Disagree
   [ ] Neutral
   [ ] Agree
   [ ] Strongly agree

6. I prefer not to express my feelings in order to avoid conflict.
   [ ] Strongly disagree
   [ ] Disagree
   [ ] Neutral
   [ ] Agree
   [ ] Strongly agree

7. My negative feelings in childhood led to being punished.
   [ ] Strongly disagree

[ ] Disagree
[ ] Neutral
[ ] Agree
[ ] Strongly agree

8. I struggle to comprehend what others are feeling.
[ ] Strongly disagree
[ ] Disagree
[ ] Neutral
[ ] Agree
[ ] Strongly agree

9. I never let on to anyone when I am angry.
[ ] Strongly disagree
[ ] Disagree
[ ] Neutral
[ ] Agree
[ ] Strongly agree

10. My strong feelings seem especially scary.
[ ] Strongly disagree
[ ] Disagree
[ ] Neutral
[ ] Agree
[ ] Strongly agree

11. I was taught to be positive at all costs.
[ ] Strongly disagree
[ ] Disagree
[ ] Neutral
[ ] Agree
[ ] Strongly agree

12. I never saw my parents argue or cry.
[ ] Strongly disagree
[ ] Disagree

[ ] Neutral
[ ] Agree
[ ] Strongly agree

13. I prefer to always be in control.
[ ] Strongly disagree
[ ] Disagree
[ ] Neutral
[ ] Agree
[ ] Strongly agree

After completing the questionnaire, take a moment to reflect on your responses. Reflect on the following questions in your journal: What patterns do you notice in your answers? How might these patterns relate to your current emotional awareness and relationships? What steps can you take to develop a healthier relationship with your emotions?

---

1. Dutton, K., (2012). The wisdom of psychopaths: What saints, spies, and serial killers can teach us about success. New York, NY, USA; Scientific American/Farrar, Straus and Giroux.

Seventeen

Attuning to Feelings

*"Mindfulness is the gateway to an awakened
life, leading to a magical, rich and quiet garden."*

— Stephen Fulder

Feelings go together with meanings

Our constant reality is one of being in continuous relationship with a procession of feelings, major and minor. Most of the time, these feelings go unacknowledged. This is not just for the reasons discussed in the previous chapter, but also because we give priority to those activities that meet our needs. Because our needs tend to be directed at some point in the future rather than in the moment, and meeting those needs is subject to time constraints, we prefer to be efficient.

This efficiency of function is a major distraction and there are other demands besides that prevent us from attending to our feelings in the moment. Consequently, we neglect at least some of our feelings most of the time. We become adept at brushing them aside, burying them, or converting them into something more acceptable.

Neglecting our feelings does not always create problems for us. However, the fact that you are struggling with GERD suggests that you have some neglected feelings that require your attention. In this regard, feelings go together with meanings. So if you have already had some success finding meaning in your GERD, you will also have begun to confront some strong feelings.

This might not always be accompanied by a shift in your physical symptoms because getting hold of these strong feelings has its own challenges. Finding ways to deal effectively with these strong feelings will be your greatest hurdle in learning to live free of GERD. But this book is all about leaping hurdles, beginning with strategies for attuning to our feelings.

Graham's story

I met Graham at a conference of the New Zealand MindBody Network. In his former life, Graham was a general practitioner who began to question his profession, the pharmaceutical industry for which he had become a patsy, and the limited value he believed he afforded his patients in overcoming their suffering.

Deeply unhappy in his role, Graham quit his practice and sought solitude in the Waipoua forest in New Zealand's far north. Outfitted with a tent for shelter but little food, Graham's intention was to be alone in nature for as long as needed to receive the inner guidance he sought to make sense of his own suffering. During his meditations, which lasted four days, Graham wanted an answer for his question, "What is the purpose of my life?"

On the fourth day, Graham's quest began to take on some clarity. As he connected deeply with the forest around him, a calm descended and he felt an opening like nothing he had experienced before. And then came his eureka moment as he was struck with the uninspired and disappointing insight that the entire point of his existence came down to a simple choice in each moment: To feel, or not to feel.

Armed with this detail, Graham packed up his tent, went home, and became deeply depressed. He remained down for the next several months as he struggled with how to *be* when the cosmos, seemingly, required so little of him.

The courage to feel

After telling me his story in person, I had the good manners to go to Graham's workshop later in the conference, which clashed with the workshop of another speaker who I had actually paid the conference fee to see. It turned out to be my good fortune that I did.

Taking my seat, I encountered immediately in Graham a person whose message to the many was delivered with the same authenticity and care he had earlier given to me in person: He spoke from his heart into my soul.

Graham proceeded to facilitate the most extraordinary experience of *feeling* in a roomful of relative strangers. His introductory message to his audience inspired the chapter *We are trained not to feel*. But it was what he got the audience to do, more so than anything he said, which transported everyone in the room away from the self-limiting thinking we all engage in to the powerful experience of wholeness that opens to us when we are courageous.

"Courage," says psychotherapist and author Stephanie Dowrick, "comes out of and expresses love." A love, she says, which reflects "a commitment to the belief that life itself is something marvelous, precious, worth having, worth living fully."[1] Without courage, we would not have the means to balance out fear and open up to life and all it throws our way. Courage sets us free.

Attuning to the person in the mirror

Attuning to our feelings is the process through which we come to acknowledge, engage with, explore and ultimately accept our feelings. Attuning to our deepest feelings, I believe, is the greatest commitment to life we can make. It requires this courage, which comes out of and expresses love, without which we are left with the ordinary and never the magical; the self-pity and denial; the white noise, and never the tranquil.

I strongly suspect that Graham helped a roomful of people open to the depth of feeling we all experienced because of his courage and the love from which it emanates. In sensing these qualities in him, we too saw these qualities in ourselves and each other.

So, when he asked us to partner up and look into this person's eyes, holding their gaze for a full two minutes, we could do so because we found the courage. And when he asked us to observe where the other person carried tension—which required us to visually scan every part of the other person's body—we were able to push through the extreme awkwardness and fear of judgment because we found the courage. And when we experienced a level of feeling toward our other that was both novel and surprising, we were able to experience the same in ourselves as we relaxed into a guided meditation to mine even greater depths of feeling only because we found the courage.

Attuning to our feelings requires us to accept our imperfections, our humanness. We are helped in this because everywhere we go, there are mirrors. When you gaze into another person's eyes, who do you see if not yourself? When you make a judgment about this person, who are you really judging? Is it true that the qualities you see in another are recognized only because you have these same qualities yourself?

As Graham discovered after four days alone in the forest—as he learned to silence his inner critic that kept him looking outward—nature became his mirror. And the more attuned he became with his essential nature, so too did he become attuned to his own essential essence. Fortunately, we do not need this level of discipline to attune to the feelings of our GERD. Our disease is a valuable mirror indeed.

Of course, you could spend thousands of dollars seeing a talk therapist or a similar amount on body-focused therapy, and this investment would certainly be worthwhile. For some people, spending time with a therapist may be essential for improving self-agency and overcoming the dysfunction that comes with the unwanted scarring of a traumatic childhood. But again, the therapist acts as a mirror for us, even if their practice assumptions sometimes do not recognize relationships as the mirrors they surely are.

Overcoming defenses: the role of the therapist

Perhaps the most difficult challenge any therapist faces is getting their clients to lower their defenses. This is a critical aspect of healing as the client begins to experience the authentic feelings that their childhood training led them to deny, suppress, or in other ways ignore. But to experience these feelings, in addition to letting down our guards, we risk an enormous vulnerability. Because in order to open to significant feelings such as anger, envy, disgust, grief, guilt, helplessness, powerlessness, shame and worthlessness, we have to allow ourselves to be vulnerable. And that requires great courage.

The therapist can help their clients in this endeavor through hosting and nurturing a relationship based on trust, respect, and unconditional positive regard. Unlike the barren, traditional relationship between therapist and client that is often depicted in the media, authentic therapeutic relationships require the therapist to mirror their own vulnerabilities.

They must display courage, warmth and stability, thereby fostering a genuine rapport with their clients. This takes time and effort. It also demands that the therapist has attended in the past to their own personal healing work and continues to attend to their self-care in the present. Not all therapeutic disciplines demand this personal undertaking; these people often struggle to be effective therapists as a result.

But the most critical factor that limits a person's progress in therapy is the therapist's inability—as a result of their training—to *see* the wholeperson. Most talk therapists see their clients above the neck and ignore the many opportunities to explore the client's—and their own—embodied stories within the same context as their spoken one. Conversely, most body-focused therapists *see* their clients from the neck down and ignore the many opportunities to explore the client's—and their own—spoken stories within the same context as their embodied one.

Overcoming defenses: becoming your own therapist

Attuning to a feeling only happens when we consciously choose to experience it first as an embodied sensation or emotion. As we experience this emotion, and its intensity grows, we might eventually give it a name in order to better relate to it. This in turn helps to bring out further aspects of our story as we learn to journey with, and accept, this significant named feeling. With the bodymind thus engaged, attuning to an emotion or embodied sensation, and naming it as a feeling we know is essentially the wholeperson approach.

Whenever we make the conscious choice to experience a feeling—however uncomfortable it makes us—we actually bypass our defenses. Within any therapeutic relationship, attuning to feelings that are emergent in the body is a large chunk of what makes good therapy effective. As someone who is seeking to overcome your own GERD using a self-healing approach, you need not be concerned about defenses as long as you are open and vulnerable to the full experience of your authentic, embodied feelings.

Defenses only work because we use them unconsciously to take us away from what makes us uncomfortable. But as long as your conscious intention is to move toward this discomfort with openness and curiosity, and without judgment, your defenses are no longer necessary. Your body is a mirror for your story and it does not lie. The diagram below illustrates this process.

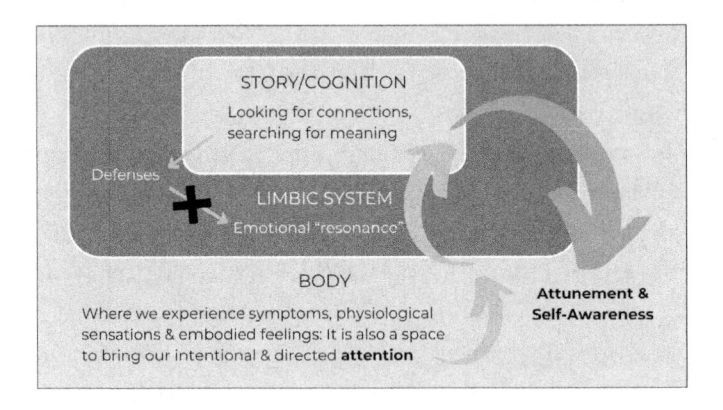

```
STORY/COGNITION
Looking for connections,
searching for meaning

Defenses

LIMBIC SYSTEM
Emotional "resonance"

BODY
Where we experience symptoms, physiological
sensations & embodied feelings: It is also a space
to bring our intentional & directed attention

Attunement &
Self-Awareness
```

Figure 17.1: *Although our story begins as a cognitive process, attuning to its associated feelings requires the full participation of our body. By being curious and intentional in the way we direct our attention to the embodied experience of emotion, we bypass our cognitive defenses and the emotion intensifies. This is the process of attunement and self-awareness.*

Transitions required for attunement and self-awareness

We can summarize the process of attunement and self-awareness as five overlapping transitions. First, our story provides entry into a deeper understanding of our GERD.

Second, story naturally engages our cognition, which is initially useful as we look for connections between our story and symptoms. Specifically we are looking to find the meaning in our personal story that precipitated our GERD around the time certain life events were occurring. However, thoughts alone will keep us stuck for the simple reason that we unconsciously withhold personal meaning when we engage our defenses.

Third, cognition is critical for our defenses, which are organized unconsciously, affect our thoughts and allow us to avoid the discomfort of our significant feelings. With our defenses up, we are unable to access the brain's limbic system, which we can think of as part of an overarching antenna that resonates with the physical sensations and emotions in our body.[2]

Fourth, when we shift our attention from our story to these embodied physical sensations and emotions, we bring these to consciousness and attune to the associated feelings. In addition to attuning to the feeling, our self-awareness improves which increases the available attention that we can give to our body.[3]

Fifth, self-awareness represents our willingness to experience our embodied feelings. As we begin to consciously attune to our feelings, the limbic system is activated and we have a heightened experience of these feelings. This may evoke memories, with subsequent re-engagement of our cognition as we seek to understand this new relationship between the feelings we just experienced and the memories evoked. Fresh insights contribute to the overarching story and the means to live free from GERD.

Attention!

The good news in this attuning process is that your body will feel more vibrant and healthy by virtue of the increased attention you give it. The bad news is that you have been trained from a young age so as not to experience the full range of feelings that we are hardwired to experience. Consequently, you are accustomed to noticing things that bring you comfort and avoiding things that cause discomfort.

The further good news, however, is that the more you consciously choose to experience your difficult feelings, the easier it becomes. By choosing consciously to experience your discomfort, you are aligning with your personal growth and healing. And you are attuning to the wisdom of your bodymind, which is not only invested in your material needs, but also your self-actualization and with it the unbounded self.

There are tools and traditions to help you better focus your attention on your body and increase your self-awareness. Meditation, Qi Gong, Tai Chi and yoga are just a few examples, but creativity is the one tool most often overlooked. So if you enjoy pottery or are a hobby mechanic, you can use your favorite creative outlet to attune to what you are feeling simply by being mindful of how your body experiences the world in the present.

Practicing mindfulness

Contrary to belief, mindfulness practice is not limited to the serious meditator who sits on their backside, with back straight and legs folded in lotus position. Mindfulness is an anytime, anywhere activity. You can practice mindfulness whether sitting or lying down, standing at the kitchen bench, walking the dog, or stopped at traffic lights.

Mindfulness is a practice that carries the energy of awareness, and involves going beyond the usual mind chatter to a concerted focus on the one activity you are engaged in. As you learn to focus your awareness on your feelings around GERD, you may begin to notice a stillness and with it fresh insight.

In a sense, giving your focused attention to your GERD feelings is the opposite of forgetfulness. This is because mindfulness helps you to attune to feelings that were present when your GERD first started, but which you were defended against and avoided due to the associated discomfort. You are simply attuning to remember, but in the present moment.

When you fully experience these feelings, this is when insights happen, remembering takes place, and healing breakthroughs occur. The concentration you exert to achieve such breakthroughs is like using a magnifying glass to focus the light of the sun.

Exercise 17.1: Mindfulness practice for attuning to feelings

This is a mindfulness exercise to help attune to your feelings. When you've finished, journal any insights.

1. **Find a comfortable position:** Start in a comfortable position, whether sitting or lying down.

2. **Begin mindful breathing:** Breathe in and out gently, noticing each in-breath and each out-breath.

3. **Become a silent observer of your breathing:** Notice how your breath becomes deeper and slower.

4. **Lengthen the pause:** Allow the pause between breaths to lengthen. Feel the silent space where thoughts are absent.

5. **Expand your awareness:** Expand your focus to your entire bodymind, paying attention to all sensations and feelings that arise.

6. **Identify tension and discomfort:** Notice any areas of tension, pain, or discomfort in your bodymind.

7. **Direct your breath:** Direct the awareness of your breath to the area of tension or discomfort. Observe how it changes.

8. **Focus on a single sensation:** Choose one sensation to concentrate on. Maintain your focus for as long as possible while breathing deeply.

9. **Allow awareness to flow:** As you focus, let your awareness move around and through the sensation. Notice any thoughts or feelings that arise.

10. **Connect with any disturbance:** If you feel disturbance or intensifying discomfort, connect with it fully instead of resisting. Observe how merging with this one sensation can lead to change within you.

11. **Practice the dance of attunement:** Recognize the evolving relationship between you and the sensation, appreciating this process as the dance of attunement.

---

1. Dowrick, S., (1997). Forgiveness and other acts of love. New York, NY, USA; W.W. Norton & Company.

2. Kelly, R., (2008). The human antenna: Reading the language of the universe in the songs of our cells. Santa Rosa, CA, USA; Energy Psychology Press.

3. Nagatomo, S., (1992). Attunement through the body. New York, NY, USA; State University of New York Press.

Eighteen

Giving Feelings a Name

The feelings wheel

Having a language for feelings is crucial for bypassing cognitive override—the defenses we employ to keep our emotions at a distance. Language helps us to articulate and confront these emotions, transforming what are unconscious sensations into conscious awareness.

The feelings wheel is a useful tool for understanding and articulating emotions, as it visually organizes feelings in a way that reveals their relationships and nuances. Unlike lists of feelings, which are commonly organized alphabetically, the feelings wheel presents feelings in a circular format. The broad categories of feelings in the center branch out into increasingly more differentiated feelings in the middle and outer layers of the wheel.

The wheel's center typically includes primary emotions that we first learn about as young children. These are the sad, bad, mad and glad feelings that are deeply rooted in psychological theories and which—in the example wheel below—are represented as joyful, sad, mad, peaceful, scared and powerful. These core feelings are universal and biologically ingrained, serving as our foundation for more complex emotional experiences that require us to articulate differentiated feelings, with the effect that we develop enhanced emotional awareness and understanding.

By using the feelings wheel, you can better navigate your own emotional landscape, learning to recognize subtle differences between feelings, and articulating your experiences more clearly.

Exercise 18.1: The wheel of feels exercise

As a brief exercise, take a close look at the feeling's wheel with the intention of identifying possible feelings associated with your GERD. Speak aloud the names of any feelings you associate with your symptoms, and which you think may be important.

Observe where the corresponding resonance is in your body. Notice in particular those feelings whose resonances are located in the region of your symptoms (e.g., stomach, chest, mouth and throat). Do these feelings help to tell your story?

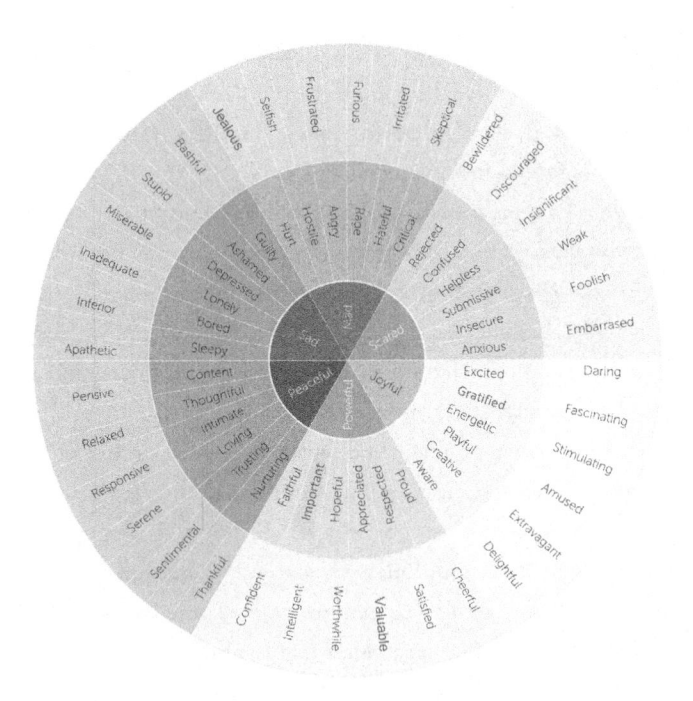

Figure 18.1: *The Feelings Wheel: Modified from an image by Thehistoryhead available at https://commons.wikimedia.org/wiki/File:The_Feelings_Wheel.png and licensed under a Creative Commons Attribution-Share Alike 4.0 International license.*

Locating your feelings

Feelings make our experiences—and our stories about them—relatable, memorable and *meaningful*. Hopefully, the feeling's wheel exercise has helped you identify some candidate feelings for your GERD and allowed you to feel a corresponding resonance in your body as you named those feelings. When we give our feelings a name and bring them back to our body, our feelings may come to symbolize our GERD in an especially meaningful way.

Consider this: The embodied *location* of a particular symptom, sensation or emotion can be a clue as to its corresponding feeling that we need to articulate.

For most people, primary emotions are easy to "locate" as we are hardwired to notice the affect in others' faces. In this sense, there is a sameness about our feelings, which we can describe in a shared context. But in another sense, our experiences of feelings are also subjective. For example, joy is universally transparent in a person's face, but one person may experience its subjective qualities in their chest and another the legs.[1] Not everyone expresses embarrassment in their cheeks, but we can recognize the affect when we see it on a person's face. Sadness is easily recognized in someone's tears, yet there is a quality and depth to our sadness that only we know. Anger is also easy to spot in a person's face, yet not everyone experiences anger in their balled-up fists.

So, when we talk about locating our feelings, it is the subjective quality of the feeling that we are most interested in. This is because we each have unique patterns—and locations—of feeling, which may change depending on the feeling's intensity and context. This is consistent with the subjective nature of the experiences through which our feelings are evoked.

Locating feelings is a prominent feature of Traditional Chinese Medicine for which the heart is the emperor of the body, the lungs hold grief, and the kidneys bear our desires and fears. William Shakespeare's use of language is especially visceral, with his life's work giving us many notable metaphors, including some that may be relevant for our GERD. Here are a few examples:

Henry V

"He which hath no stomach to this fight,
Let him depart: His passport shall be made,
And crowns for convoy put into his purse:
We would not die in that man's company
That fears his fellowship to die with us."

    Henry V rallies his soldiers to show courage and unity. A person with "no stomach to this fight" not only lacks courage, he also shows disloyalty to Henry's command. The stomach is a metaphor for courage and loyalty.

A Midsummer Night's Dream

"For as a surfeit of the sweetest things
The deepest loathing to the stomach brings,
Or as the heresies that men do leave
Are hated most of those they did deceive
So thou, my surfeit and my heresy,
Of all be hated, but the most of me."

    Lysander appears to be saying to his lover—the sleeping Hermia—that eating too many sweet things makes people sick to their stomachs. But he also acknowledges that no one hates the mistakes that people make more so than the one who made them. Hermia then is Lysander's sweet mistake who he now hates as a form of self-protection, with the stomach a metaphor for self-loathing.

Othello

"'Tis not a year or two shows a man.
They are all but stomachs, and we all but food.
They eat us hungrily, and when they are full,
They belch us."

Emilia uses her stomach metaphor to express her resentment of men and the abuse and mistreatment of women they are responsible for.

Julius Caesar

"This rudeness is a sauce to his good wit,
Which gives men stomach to digest his words
With better appetite."

Cassius uses this metaphor to explain that Casca is not the dimwit he is made out to be, but rather chooses his words to manipulate others' hunger for his ideas. The stomach is a metaphor for tolerance and manipulation.

The Tempest

"You cram these words into mine ears
Against the stomach of my sense."

Alonso tells Gonzalo that he has no desire to hear Gonzalo's words. The stomach is a metaphor for desire.

The Taming of the Shrew

"Fall to them as you find your stomach serves you
No profit grows where is no pleasure ta'en."

Tranio advises Lucentio that there is no profit where there is no pleasure; the stomach being a metaphor for pleasure.

Amplifying your feelings

Giving your GERD-related feelings a name and bringing them back to your body provides the means through which your relationship with these feelings can grow. Ultimately, it is through this relationship that we learn the value of these feelings despite the discomfort that they might bring.

Even the toxic shame that blights the life of every human being in one way or another has a role in bringing us to our authentic goals and values. Strong feelings like shame are symbols for self-awareness and self-knowledge. Once we begin to understand their value in our lives, we can transform our feelings into a force for authentic empowerment.

This transformation occurs when we amplify our relationship with the feelings in question. This is akin to developing a relationship with another person, a process involving attraction, curiosity, mutual discovery, generosity, showing tolerance and restraint, opening to vulnerability, and practicing fidelity.

In her book *Forgiveness and Other Acts of Love*, Stephanie Dowrick uses the term "fidelity" to refer to the deep commitment to love and truthfulness required for healthy relationships.[2] Fidelity encompasses more than just loyalty; it requires a willingness to be honest, to engage deeply with others, and to conduct ourselves with integrity. In this context, fidelity is a binding force that nourishes relationships, but it could just as easily describe the relationship we have with our own feelings. By showing fidelity toward our feelings, we are able to walk and talk our truth, fostering an environment where difficult conversations emphasize empathy, perspective-taking, and understanding. To shun a feeling for any reduction in discomfort is to risk the greater rewards of the relationship.

There are some simple ways to enhance our relationship with GERD-related feelings without feeling unsafe. In addition to identifying the feeling's location, we can use our curiosity and imagination to give a feeling a color, texture, smell, temperature, sound, voice, flavor, or any other quality. If you do not have a name for your feelings, then describing them with one or more of these qualities is a great way of enhancing your relationship. These qualities may be symbolic in their own right and thus may hold the key to raising awareness of the all-important meaning of your disease.

Your SUDS score

The Subjective Units of Distress Scale (SUDS) is a simple psychological measurement tool that we can use to assess any distress around our symptoms and their related feelings. Dr. Joseph Wolpe developed the SUDS in the 1960s as part of his work in behavior therapy to enable his patients to give a simple self-report of their emotional distress in response to specific triggers.

SUDS is now widely used in cognitive and trauma-focused therapies, and is often used for research purposes. As its name suggests, the scale is based on the idea that emotional distress is subjective. By allowing individuals to rate their distress on a scale from 0 (no distress) to 10 (maximum distress), SUDS acknowledges our personal experience and helps us to track any changes as we process the distress. This makes it a practical tool for monitoring progress.

Overall, the SUDS is a straightforward yet effective tool for self-reporting distress levels, facilitating a deeper understanding of emotional experiences and aiding therapeutic interventions.

Exercise 18.2: Determining your SUDS score

Your symptoms reflect your own feelings, which uniquely reflect your own struggles. Ask yourself: What is the part of your GERD—the subjective aspect that no one else can see or measure but you—that causes you to suffer most?

Whether this aspect comes to you immediately or not, imagine it can be scored from 0–10, with ten being the most distress imaginable and zero being no distress at all. For now, remember this number. This is your SUDS score.

In the next chapter, we are going to work on bringing your SUDS score to zero.

1. I once conducted this exercise with a group of Year 5 (Grade 4) students, and they quickly grasped that the experience of a simple feeling like joy can vary dramatically from one person to another. They effortlessly connected feelings of joy to different parts of their bodies, revealing that each child's perception of joy was uniquely their own.

2. Dowrick, S., (1997). Forgiveness and other acts of love. New York, NY, USA; W.W. Norton & Company.

NINETEEN

Accepting and Reframing Feelings through Energy Psychology

"When we stop opposing reality, action becomes simple, fluid, kind, and fearless."

— Byron Katie

What if the ground of reality—the foundational substance from which everything emerges—is not matter but Consciousness: That there is no thing that is not Consciousness?

Energy psychology unlocks the power within you

Get ready to embark on a transformative journey where psychology meets the remarkable universe of energy! For a while now Energy Psychology has been quietly revolutionizing the way we understand and heal the wholeperson, offering fresh insights that tap into the subtle energies influencing our emotions and behaviors. Imagine releasing emotional blocks and, in the process, transforming your psychological *and* physical well-being through innovative techniques that tap into your energy field. With Energy Psychology, you are not just a passive participant in your healing journey, you become an empowered co-creator in a self-healing process.

When we combine psychology with energy, we gain more than the sum of its parts: We join a growing awareness that unites an ancient wisdom with our modern understanding of a MindBody or meaning-based story approach to healing, and discover how to unleash our true potential to live our best life.

As we dive into the exciting realm of Energy Psychology, it is instructive to acknowledge the diverse array of modalities that have emerged from inside and outside psychotherapeutic practice over the past three decades. From Thought Field Therapy and the Tapas Acupressure Technique to Seemorg Matrix Work and Dynamic Energetic Healing, these innovative approaches have redefined how we address emotional, psychological and physical challenges. Additionally, practices like Biofield Integration, Hypnotic Language, Eye Movement Desensitization and Reprocessing (EMDR), and Integrative Energy and Spiritual Therapy offer unique pathways to healing and self-discovery.[1] Among these transformative tools, Emotional Freedom Techniques (EFT) is a powerful modality for releasing emotional blockages and fostering lasting well-being.[2]

EFT for deeper healing of our disturbed "I Am"

EFT is a simple and easy-to-learn tool through which you can quickly *accept* and release the feelings that make up your disturbed "I Am." Having released these feelings, EFT is also useful for reframing your experiences to promote deeper healing, deal more effectively with future challenging situations, maintain a constructive and productive mindset, provide new strategies for coping, increase empowerment through greater self-agency, and improve relationships. Reframing helps to integrate emotional processing within its broadest context, leading to a more balanced and fulfilling perspective on our life experiences.

Combining eastern acupressure with western cognitive and exposure therapy as it does, EFT is neither a body-focused nor mind-focused tool. Instead, it is a tool for the bodymind that does not require any mainstream assumptions about what body and mind are. EFT can be applied equally to emotional, psychological and physical issues, and even spiritual issues. You get to decide where, when and how you use EFT; it is your own imagination that determines its limits. EFT is a remarkable tool that when applied to your GERD story and feelings will likely surprise you with how effective it is.[3]

Why feelings require our acceptance

Disturbances in our sense of "I Am" can be expressed through our embodied emotions, thoughts, behaviors, learning difficulties, interpersonal relationships, self-esteem, coping mechanisms, sleep patterns, performance, decision-making, body language, mood, and physical symptoms. These disturbances not only manifest in various aspects of our lives, but they also highlight the interconnectedness of our feelings and experiences: Our experiences shape our feelings, and our feelings shape our experiences. This creates an ever-unfolding cycle of interactions among the many different elements that drive our reality, including our sense perceptions, memories, expectations, core beliefs, and intuitions.

Bringing greater self-agency to our experiences requires a shift in the way we respond to our feelings. Instead of resisting or defending against them, we must accept our feelings—however unpleasant—as integral facets of our human experience. Acceptance allows us to navigate the complexities of our internal landscape, and persist in our navigation even when we are lost. Acceptance offers us emotional resilience and self-awareness. It promotes healthier relationships with self and others. Ultimately, by accepting our feelings, we are empowered to break the cycle of disturbances and cultivate a more authentic sense of "I am."

Acceptance then is a life-affirming action that ensures we are able to create the best possible reality for ourselves and others. This includes changing our experience of GERD along with any other illnesses we may be struggling with.

It may seem incongruous to accept the very feelings that are at the root of our distress; isn't that like inviting the wolf for supper when the wolf sees us as its meal ticket?

To ask this question at all is to approach a much larger question that asks, *Why do we suffer?* In other words, the question holds universal significance with meaning beyond our individual circumstances. I offer a personal perspective on this at the end of the book. You will have your own perspective too.

The paradox of healing

There is a related question that we can ponder more readily: Why would we stand alongside our enemy let alone embrace them as a kindred spirit?

Is it because all our efforts at resisting and besting GERD have amounted to nothing but more pain? Is it because we learn to see in our enemy something that we recognize in ourselves? Is it because we understand that to accept ourselves, we also need to accept the enemy who brought us pain and suffering?

This is the paradox of healing: That which we resist persists; and that which we accept comes to pass.

In the context of healing, our resistance *is* the struggle—the more we fight against our pain, the more entrenched it can become, amplifying the very feelings we seek to avoid to the point where we can no longer ignore them.

Conversely, when we adopt the mindset of acceptance—a state of "no effort"—we begin to experience our feelings without judgment. This does not mean that we passively resign to our suffering; rather, acceptance is the en**cour**-**age**ment that we need to be present with our feelings, acknowledging them as vital agents of our human experience.[4] In this space of non-resistance, we cultivate self-compassion and openness, which are more than useful partners in our transformation.

In this light, acceptance is the doorway to healing; it is the opening in the veil of our consciousness. Far from being passive, the "no effort" of our acceptance is a bountiful and active stance that requires our attention if we are to allow our true nature to unfold. It is in this acceptance that we find clarity and healing—transformative changes that arise effortlessly when we stop resisting what *is*. The paradox reveals that healing is not a destination to be reached through sheer willpower, but a journey of gentle surrender and profound meaning.

Of course, it is okay to have doubts that GERD will exploit our acceptance as weakness. But isn't the possibility of our healing a better risk than the certainty of our struggle?

A simple EFT protocol

EFT involves the gentle tapping of specific meridian points on the body while focusing on a particular emotional issue or distressing thought. The process aims to reduce negative emotions, relieve stress, and promote well-being by balancing the body's natural energy system. EFT has been used successfully for various hard-to-treat issues, such as anxiety, depression, phobias and trauma, and is often considered a self-help tool for emotional healing.[5,6] EFT can be a powerful way to process your GERD story and its associated distress. Here's a step-by-step process:

Step 1: Identify your problem

Start by clearly defining the issue you want to resolve. Instead of saying something broad like, "I want to get rid of my acid reflux disease," think more deeply about your experience. Reflect on the specific feelings and sensations that arise. This could mean exploring emotional connections, physical sensations, or any underlying aspects of your story.

Step 2: Rate your distress

If you have yet to do so (see: *Exercise 18.2: Determining your SUDS score* from the previous *chapter*), rate your current level of distress using the Subjective Units of Distress (SUDS) scale from 0 to 10. A score of 0 indicates no distress, while 10 represents maximum distress. This rating will help track your progress.

Step 3: Create your problem statement

A well-formulated problem statement will enhance the effectiveness of your EFT experience. Include the following elements:

1. **Feeling:** Name a specific feeling related to your GERD, even if it's a creative or unique term that resonates with you.

2. **Location:** Identify where in your body you experience this feeling. This could be your stomach, throat, chest, or somewhere else.

3. **Subjective details:** Add any personal meanings or experiences tied to your suffering. What does this discomfort represent for you?

4. **SUDS:** Include your SUDS score from Step 2 in your statement.

Example problem statement

Here's an example of a problem statement based on David's experience of GERD in *Working with symbols*: "I'm hungry for success and I feel this as a burning need in my stomach and it's a 9 out of 10."

Or, here's an example based on my own experience of GERD: "I have this feeling in my stomach that I'm not enough and it's an 8 out of 10."

Step 4: Craft your opening and acceptance statement

In EFT, we can use the phrase "even though" to begin our problem statement on a neutral note, followed by the specifics of our experience. We always need to end with an acceptance statement, which relates to the all important healing paradox. You can use "I accept myself completely" or create a variation that feels genuinely accepting for you.

Example statement

Here's David's statement: "Even though I'm hungry for success and I feel this as a burning need in my stomach and it's a 9 out of 10, I'm okay with myself."

And here's my statement: "Even though I have this feeling in my stomach that I'm not enough and it's an 8 out of 10, I accept myself completely."

Step 5: Fine-tune your statement

Feel free to adjust the length of your problem statement based on intuition:

- **Short example:** "I feel shame in my stomach at a 9 out of 10."

- **Long example:** "I have this gray, icky feeling at the back of my throat that crawls out of my stomach, and it's a 7 out of 10."

Step 6: Process each statement separately

If your statement is lengthy or covers multiple feelings, break it down into manageable parts. Tackle each statement one at a time, ensuring each includes an acceptance phrase. For example:

1. "I feel this gray, icky sensation at the back of my throat, and it's a 7 out of 10. I accept myself completely."

2. "It crawls out of my stomach and it's a 5. I accept myself completely."

By structuring your use of EFT in this way, you create a focused pathway toward understanding and processing your GERD symptoms. Engage your creativity, and feel free to modify your statements to best express your unique experiences. Remember, the real goal of EFT is not simply to relieve symptoms, but to *find* yourself in the "no effort" space of acceptance.

Setup and reminder phrases for EFT

Now that you have your problem statement(s), it is time to integrate them into the EFT protocol. This involves using tapping pressure to activate acupressure points on your hand, face, and chest while speaking your problem statement aloud or internally.

At first, this may seem unusual, but as you notice its effects, EFT will soon become second nature. We unconsciously stimulate these acupressure points when we rub our eyes, blow our noses, or scratch our heads—this practice simply brings those natural instincts into conscious awareness.

Using EFT to "set up" your problem statement

To activate each acupressure point through tapping, follow these simple steps:

1. **Karate chop point (KC):** Begin by tapping the karate chop point of your non-dominant hand with the first and second fingers of your dominant hand. This point is located on the outer edge of your hand, where you would strike if breaking a plank of wood (**Figure 19.1**).

2. **Speak your statement:** While tapping the KC point, repeat your problem statement, including SUDS score and acceptance statement.

Example

While tapping the KC point, you might say: "Even though I'm hungry for success and I feel this as a burning need in my stomach and it's a 9 out of 10, I'm okay with myself." Or, "Even though I have this feeling in my stomach that I'm not enough and it's an 8 out of 10, I accept myself completely."

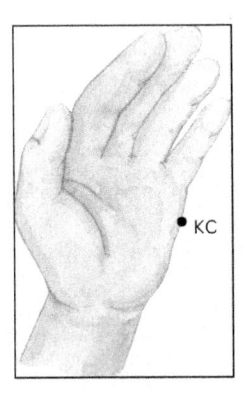

Figure 19.1: *Tap continuously on the "set up" or KC point using the 1st and 2nd fingers of your dominant hand while speaking aloud—or in your mind—the entire problem statement, including SUDS score and acceptance statement.*

Using EFT to remind yourself of the problem

After you have completed the set up, there is no need to repeat the entire problem statement during the rest of the EFT process. Instead, you can use shorter reminder phrases while tapping on the remaining points (**Figure 19.2**).

Reminder phrase

Select a phrase that captures the essence of your problem statement. This phrase should focus on the feeling you have identified and now aim to accept, without including your SUDS score or acceptance statement.

Examples of reminder statements

For David: "This hunger for success," or "This burning need in my stomach."
For myself: "This feeling in my stomach that I'm not enough."

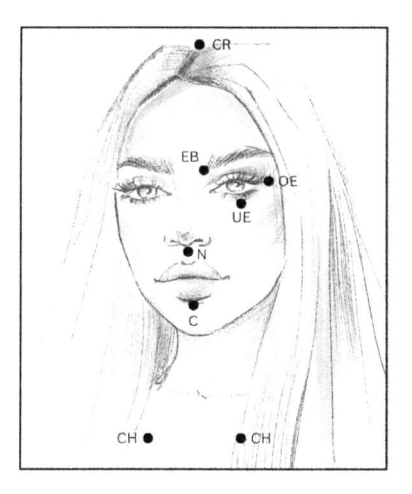

Figure 19.2: *Tap on each of the reminder points in turn while speaking aloud (or in your mind) the reminder statement.*

Tapping sequence

As you go through the tapping sequence, focus on your reminder phrase. Here are the points you will tap:

1. **Crown (CR):** Tap the crown of your head.

2. **Eyebrow (EB):** Tap the inside end of the eyebrow, where the bridge of the nose begins.

3. **Outer eye (OE):** Tap on the bony ridge of the eye socket, immediately to the outer side of the eye.

4. **Under eye (UE):** Tap on the bony ridge underneath the eye.

5. **Nose (N):** Tap just below the nose, at the top of the philtrum.

6. **Chin (C):** Tap immediately beneath your bottom lip.

7. **Chest (CH):** Tap the hollows beside the collarbone. Use your thumb and first two fingers, splayed apart to form a gun shape.

8. **Under arm (UA):** Tap in the hollow of your armpit, aligned with the nipples. You may find tenderness at this point, as it is a lymphatic drainage site.

9. **Under nipple (UN):** Tap between two ribs, about a hand's width below the nipple.

Tapping on each of these points sequentially while using your reminder phrase constitutes one full round of EFT. Typically, spend two to three seconds tapping each point, but trust your intuition—you may feel moved to linger longer on specific areas if needed.

If you haven't had a chance to try EFT yet, consider doing so now before proceeding to the next section.

Getting your SUDS score down

Take a moment to revisit your SUDS score after doing one round of EFT. Has it decreased, increased, or stayed the same?

When our SUDS score goes up

While we always aim for our SUDS score to drop, sometimes our distress can increase when we are addressing important issues. There are several possible reasons for this.

First, as we engage with our emotional distress, we may bring unresolved feelings to the surface. This increased distress can signify that we are touching on core issues that need our closer attention. Second, tapping can enhance our awareness of underlying emotions or beliefs that may have previously been buried. Confronting these deeper issues may result in a temporary rise in distress with our increased awareness. Third, as we process our issues, our view of the situation often changes, leading to heightened feelings. This can lead to a higher SUDS score initially, but it also signifies that we are moving closer to understanding and resolving a specific, underlying issue. Finally, much like a physical detoxification, emotional processing can stir up difficult feelings. Any rise in SUDS score may be part of the "cleansing" that occurs when we confront difficult but necessary issues for our healing.

Ultimately, a rise in your SUDS score can be a sign of progress in your emotional journey, indicating that you are working through significant issues. Consistent effort will help you to move toward a resolution.

When our SUDS score doesn't go down

Sometimes our SUDS score doesn't decrease as expected. This is especially true for complex and stubborn issues like GERD, which often have multiple underlying aspects. For instance, while working through complex feelings, new aspects may arise, such as memories, shifts in sensations, or unexpected insights. These moments are opportunities to go deeper into your experience.

In my own journey with GERD, I discovered several important layers that influenced my feelings. For example, I recalled a distressing memory from childhood when my mother laughed at my offer to help with household finances during a tough time (see: *Identifying specific memories*). Recognizing this connection allowed me to craft a more focused problem statement:

"Even though I felt a sinking feeling in my stomach when my mother said we may lose our home and laughed at my offer to help, I accept myself completely."

This statement opened up additional embodied emotions, which I related to a feeling of inadequacy. I continued to engage with my emotions, leading to a realization: "I never have enough."

This new understanding prompted me to explore my feelings of grief and lack—acknowledging not just financial insecurity but also emotional neglect as a child. I transformed this insight into another problem statement: "Even though I never have enough; as a child I lacked nourishment, emotional security, and warmth from the people I looked to for love, I accept myself completely."

As I tapped through these evolving statements, I acknowledged feelings of shame associated with my experiences. Each round of EFT allowed me to further address these feelings, leading to a drop in my SUDS score. Eventually, I reached the point where my SUDS score was zero, reflecting a significant release of these long-held feelings.

Practical steps to lowering stubborn SUDS scores

1. **Revisit and refine your statements:** After your initial rounds of EFT, take note of any new feelings or memories that emerge. Use these insights to create new, specific problem statements for your next tapping session.

2. **Acknowledge all layers:** Understand that emotional issues often have multiple layers. If feelings intensify, recognize this as a chance to delve deeper into the root causes.

3. **Tap on new insights:** Whenever new layers of emotion or thought arise, include them in your tapping statements. For example, if you

realize that your feelings of insecurity are connected to childhood experiences, add those specifics to your problem statement.

4. **Be patient and persevere:** Emotional healing can be a gradual process. Stay committed, even if your SUDS score fluctuates. Trust that working through these complexities will lead to a resolution.

By addressing the multifaceted nature of your feelings and embracing the process of exploration, you can ultimately reduce stubborn SUDS scores and facilitate healing. Your journey may reveal unexpected insights about yourself, just as mine did, potentially transforming your relationship with GERD and your emotional, psychological and physical well-being.

Reframes

Reframing is a powerful step in the EFT process, particularly after you have successfully lowered your SUDS score to 2 or below. This is the moment where you can transform previously limiting beliefs into positive affirmations that support your healing and growth. If your experience with GERD has revealed inadequacy, scarcity, worthlessness, anxiety, shame, or other significant feelings, this is your chance to reframe not only the feelings, but also the core beliefs our feelings give rise to.

For example, if you have identified a core belief like "I am not enough," consider flipping that around. You might substitute it with a healthier affirmation, such as "I have more than enough for myself and others." This shift not only helps alleviate the impact of those negative feelings but also empowers you to face challenges with a renewed sense of self-worth.

Next time you encounter a situation that triggers a certain feeling, remind yourself of your new positive belief. With practice, you will find that your emotional resilience increases, reducing your reliance on physical symptoms like GERD to prompt you to reflect on your overall well-being. Wholeness is experienced in the moment; the key is to keep reminding yourself of this truth.

Take a moment to think about how you might reframe your own GERD experience. This process may involve exploring the feelings associated with it more deeply, uncovering how something that once felt destructive can also serve as a catalyst for positive change in your life.

Exploring your feelings

Understanding your feelings is crucial for effective reframing. Here are some practical tips to help you delve deeper into your feelings for powerful reframes:

1. **Assign a color to your feeling:** Name your feeling and describe its location. Then, give it a color and incorporate this into your problem statement and reminder phrase. During your next round of EFT, observe any changes in the color and feeling that arise. Ask yourself, "What does this color remind me of?"

2. **Identify the texture of your feeling:** Describe the feeling using textures, such as "hard and stony," "lumpy," or "soft and moist." Include these descriptions in your statements. Reflect on their significance by asking, "What does this texture remind me of?"

3. **Explore additional descriptions:** Go beyond just naming and locating your feelings. Consider questions like, "What is its age?" or "Who does it remind me of and why?" Imagining the feeling as a person with a face may also provide insights into its nature.

4. **Refer to your journal:** Look back over your journal entries for ideas that can serve as problem statements. Trust your creativity and intuition while using EFT—they can guide you in uncovering deeper insights about your feelings.

By dedicating time to reflect on and reframe your feelings, you pave the way for a more positive outlook on your experiences with GERD. This process transforms what may have been negative influences into empowering beliefs that support your journey to healing and wholeness.

1. Gallo, F. P., (ed.), (2002). Energy psychology in psychotherapy: A comprehensive source book. New York, NY, USA; W. W. Norton & Company, Inc.

2. Of all the self-help tools that have been brought into the public consciousness, EFT is the most freely accessible, easy to learn, and among the most controversial. With its basis in eastern acupressure and western cognitive behavioral science, EFT is a blend of ideas that are both esoteric and open source. EFT's principal innovator, Gary Craig, long ago set aside profit motives for EFT's blended ideas and instead offers plenty of free advice, tutorials and videos at www.palaceofpossibilities.com. Another website, www.eftuniverse.com also offers a range of useful and free resources. These include a comprehensive how-to EFT manual. EFT is simple to learn and even gain a level of mastery without having to pay someone to teach you. One of the downsides of EFT is that its use does not translate readily into the relational setting of high-quality talk therapy. Even if you do decide to go to therapy, EFT is fantastic for your between-visit homework!

3. Feinstein, D., Eden, D., & Craig, G., (2005). The promise of energy psychology: Revolutionary tools for dramatic personal change. New York, NY, USA; JP Tarcher/Penguin.

4. Zukav, G., & Francis, L., (2001). The heart of the soul: Emotional awareness. New York, NY, USA; Simon & Schuster.

5. Church, D., Stapleton, P., Vasudevan, A., & O'Keefe, T., (2022). Clinical EFT as an evidence-based practice for the treatment of psychological and physiological conditions: A systematic review. *Frontiers in Psychology*, 10(13): 951451.

6. Craig, G., (2008). EFT for PTSD (posttraumatic stress disorder). Fulton, CA, USA; Energy Psychology Press.

Twenty

Feelings as Connection

One man's medicine

Earlier, I introduced the idea of feelings as communication. Whether it is the feeling of hunger as an infant, joy as a playful child, or frustration as a parent, we learn through a combination of innate behavior and experience to communicate what we are feeling. In this way, we use the qualities of being in a relationship with anyone else to satisfy our needs.

Communicating our feelings is a lifetime endeavor and does not stop during periods of isolation or withdrawal. We simply find other things—such as toys, work and addictions—through which to meet our needs. But there is something much more to feelings, which is exemplified in this next anecdote.

During his lifetime, Dr. Archie Cochrane made a valuable contribution to evidence-based medicine when he advocated for the use of randomized clinical trials to improve our understanding of the efficacy and safety of medical interventions. A database was set up in his name. Today, any clinician wanting information about a drug or other medical intervention can search the database for up-to-date information.

Now I would not normally trouble you with a story about evidence-based medicine and the man who pushed for it except for the fact that the Cochrane Database and Dr. Archie Cochrane have been highly influential in modern medical thinking. Even then I would not trouble you with this detail, but for a slip of fate that did not hold Dr. Cochrane's attention until later in life. If it did,

I speculate, Dr. Cochrane's contribution to medicine could have looked quite different and we might not be as slow as we have been to explore our innate need for connection through the lens of our disease.

The slip of fate I refer to relates to Dr. Cochrane's experiences of working as a medical officer while a captured medic during World War II. Consider the following excerpt from his autobiography, *One Man's Medicine*:[1]

"*Another event at Elsterhorst had a marked effect on me. The Germans dumped a young Soviet prisoner in my ward late one night. The ward was full, so I put him in my room as he was moribund and screaming and I did not want to wake the ward. I examined him. He had obvious gross bilateral cavitation and a severe pleural rub. I thought the latter was the cause of the pain and the screaming. I had no morphia, just aspirin, which had no effect.*

I felt desperate. I knew very little Russian then and there was no one in the ward who did. I finally instinctively sat down on the bed and took him in my arms, and the screaming stopped almost at once. He died peacefully in my arms a few hours later. It was not the pleurisy that caused the screaming but loneliness. It was a wonderful education about the care of the dying. I was ashamed of my misdiagnosis and kept the story secret."

The bridge of connection

This anecdote has remained with me for years. It exemplifies that the most basic drive we have as human beings is for connection. We never lose this need, even in our dying moments. In this drive for connection, it is our feelings that provide the bridge, whether that feeling is of fear, pain, love, or something else.

Our pain might take us to the doctor, whereas our love might take us to the chocolatier. In both examples, the role of the doctor or chocolatier is not to validate our feelings like Dr. Cochrane did for the dying Russian soldier. Instead, they provide us with material evidence of the feeling through which we seek to build a connection. From the doctor, the evidence of our feeling could be a prescription for drugs, or even the drugs themselves. From the chocolatier, the evidence of our feeling comes from chocolates.

Continuing with these examples, we can think of the drugs or chocolates as transitional objects through which we attach our feelings in order to better explore them. We might even say that these objects appear to *speak* our feelings. They help us onto the bridge of connection, but not yet over it.

Take the example of the doctor's drugs: These have become the transitional objects of our pain. In this case, the attempt at connection is with self and occurs when we take the drug. If the drug is effective at numbing our symptoms, the feeling of pain remits and a normal connection with self resumes. If the pain was to return, however, we might become dependent on the drug for ongoing relief. Any connection with self is accordingly short-lived.

Taking the example of chocolate as a transitional object, we are validated in our feeling of love only when our suitor receives the symbol of our affection in a way that reciprocates what we feel. If our suitor does not return our affection, the feeling of love is not validated and the connection we sought remains unfulfilled. On the other hand, a reciprocal feeling of love provides an opportunity to explore a mutual connection in greater depth.

The truth of our humanity is that we all want a shared connection. Thus, we want to live and laugh together, love and express joy together, grieve and remain together. In this common purpose, our invention of entertainment like sport and theater takes on new meaning when we think of them as vessels for connection. When connection in the rest of our life is uncertain or transient, we might look to our favorite sports team or theater company to give us a shared experience of the joy or despair that are integral to our goal of uniting against a common foe.

As humanity continues to unfold, the ways in which we seek connection may well change and become even more transitory. But our basic drive for connection will always remain.

Normal versus disordered attachment

Every human being once experienced life inside their mother's womb—the original *home* of our creation and connection. As long as the fetus remains in the womb, its needs for connection, growth and development are readily met. Although protected from the outside world, the fetus is already learning to feel what its mother feels. Birth comes as a shock to the newborn, but the connection with its mother continues seamlessly if she is able to provide suitable care. The mother is more likely to be successful in this aim if she feels cared for herself.

It may be that the mother returns to work soon after the infant's birth. This can be a traumatic separation for the infant, but any long-term impact is lessened as long as the infant is permitted to form a *secure attachment base* with another caring adult.[2] Optimally, this adult has their own needs readily met and they come from a secure attachment base themselves.

Providing such a stable base for the infant requires a long-term commitment. Along its journey to becoming a resilient individual, the infant must negotiate many microtraumas. These include teething, weaning, toilet training, and the discomfort of its mother's absences, as well as hunger, wetness, coldness, scolding and the usual early childhood hurts.

When each of these microtraumas is met with the certainty of emotional security, healthy individuation occurs. This does not require perfection from the child's primary caregiver. Rather, the child's primary attachment need only be good enough.

Normal attachment that leads to healthy individuation occurs in around 75% to 85% of the general population. But the sad reality for at least 15% to 25% of the general population and at least 65% of the prison population is that their early childhood caregiver was unable to provide the secure attachment base that the child needed to thrive.[3] The resulting attachment disorder has serious potential consequences, including poor emotional development and reasoning, learning and behavior problems, socialization difficulties, coercive sexual behavior, and a high risk of mental illness, addiction and physical disease as an adult.[4,5,6]

There is no single entry point into the profound hurt of attachment disorder. However, it is important to note that the routine absence of emotional security in a child's life cannot be overcome just because their material needs are met. Attachment disorder does not discriminate generally in who it impacts. Although it is more common with poverty, attachment disorder occurs regardless of the socioeconomic status of the child's family and reflects society's wider attitudes toward motherhood, fatherhood and the support we give caregivers of children.[7]

Curiously, attachment disorder does discriminate along gender lines, with boys more likely than girls to demonstrate externalizing behaviors such as anger and aggression. In contrast, girls are more likely than boys to show internalizing behaviors such as anxiety, depression and eating disorders. Compared with their securely attached peers, children with disordered attachment have a greater likelihood for physical disease, as well as impaired psychological and social functioning that extends into adulthood.[8]

The feelings of attachment

Attachment disorder provides incontrovertible evidence of the need for connection in early childhood and what happens when this need is unmet. But to understand the basis for a child's wounding when connection is absent, we need to consider the role of affect, emotions and feelings once more.

Newborn infants (as for adults) recognize their needs according to the sensations of their bodies. The infant's nervous system is aroused to a particular sensation—for example discomfort—and the infant displays the accompanying affect as a primitive form of emotion through its facial muscles, body language and cry. The caregiver's ability to identify and respond to each message or emotion provides the infant with important feedback. These exchanges give the infant its earliest lessons in regulating its own emotions.

Critically, the caregiver's own facial expressions, body language, voice, scent, touch and even their heart rhythms provide cues to the infant's inner discovery of self. What the caregiver *shows*, the infant uses mirror neurons in its brain to model for itself. It is through these sensory inputs it receives from the caregiver that the infant is able to make sense of its world. What the caregiver feels, the infant learns too. In the infant's early comprehension, the caregiver and it are one and the same.

This empathetic modeling is the path to more nuanced empathy, as well as self-esteem, restraint, generosity, tolerance, and our commitment to love, truthfulness and integrity. Such empathetic sharing of feelings provides us with a sense of place and belonging in the world that is vital for our personal and communal well-being; our sense of connection and interconnectedness.

In the same way that an enriched connection in early childhood provides a foundation for enriched socialization opportunities and well-being, a poor connection unfortunately sets the scene for poor socialization and well-being. Imagine an infant or young child who experiences prolonged periods of discomfort, often alone, without relief. And when the relief does come, any corresponding cues from the caregiver involve anger, grief or some other signal that threatens the infant's already compromised safety and security needs. How might we expect such an infant to develop?

Each child and each child's situation is of course unique. But in general terms, an infant (up to one year old) might experience embodied sensations that we might think of as emptiness, coldness and helplessness. A toddler whose chief aim is to know self through otherness might experience embodied sensations that we could think of as powerlessness, shame, anger and self-disgust. A preschool aged child might build on these with embodied feelings of hopelessness, loneliness, isolation, despair, and worthlessness. At any stage the child will almost certainly experience feelings of anxiety and grief.

Reconnection as healing

In the absence of the positive feelings that we normally associate with connection—care, compassion, appreciation, gratitude, joy, love—our drive for connection is not diminished. On the contrary, our drive for connection is just as strong. But instead of being informed by positive feelings, this drive will be informed by any of the many negative feelings.

In turn, this can create an expectation for only having negative experiences. For many people—and especially those with attachment disordered childhoods—constant negative feelings and their associated thoughts manifest in a vicious cycle of negative experiences. Such people may still connect with others in meaningful ways. Many live productive lives.

But unresolved traumas and losses may lead to a person sabotaging important relationships in order to follow the same (mal)adaptive paths that they learned to take in early childhood in order to feel safe. Another person may be very controlling in their relationships, lacking empathy, and using grandiose behaviors and manipulative tactics to have their needs met. Yet another person may appear needy in relationships, yet be passive in terms of meeting others' needs. Many people who have experienced significant early trauma develop personality disorders. If unrecognized and untreated, such disorders can be especially detrimental to achieving prosocial outcomes.

The patterns of feeling associated with such maladaptive personality traits and their associated behaviors are no less meaningful than the predominantly positive feeling patterns that we see in healthy attachment relationships. It is important to realize that all feelings and the behaviors that they determine are a form of communication, connection and—in the case of negative patterns—our attempts at reconnection.

Healing, then, involves identifying and working with our negative feeling states and the underlying traumas that they represent to reconnect with self and the innate human potential that we are all capable of unleashing.

Persistent negative feelings: A time for change

Imagine yourself reacting harshly to a loved one's comment, or think of a past situation where a friend offered their constructive criticism, but instead of appreciating their perspective you responded defensively. Perhaps you can recall a minor disagreement with a partner that escalated into an argument, or feeling an unexplained irritation toward a colleague's enthusiasm?

There is no better way of identifying our negative feeling states than when we are in relationship with another. Across our different relationships, our recurrent negative feelings and the behaviors that they produce can become obvious to us when we recognize that the person opposite us mirrors our behavior.

If we show aggression, they might recoil or become aggressive in return. If we show helplessness, we might unwittingly provoke their anxiety or, if they are well-adjusted, an empathetic response. If we show shame, we could provoke disgust or rejection, whereas a more balanced person might show tolerance or even compassion.

If we want to change for the better—and our recurrent negative feelings are the cue that change is a good idea—it is helpful to understand that the negative feelings that we express encode vital information from our bodies. This could be information about past traumas, losses and other painful experiences. When the feelings we communicate make someone uncomfortable, including ourselves, this presents an opportunity to discover something about our past that needs to be brought into awareness.

When the time is right, we can safely revisit these past experiences with a view toward: Processing the content and context of the experiences; finding the meaning that is waiting to be unearthed; releasing the negative feelings to resolve past traumas and hurts; and reframing these stories to create authentic power for ourselves and others.

Identifying early childhood trauma

Understanding ourselves as adults often means revisiting our childhoods, which can uncover complex emotions and experiences that shape who we are today. For many, recognizing the impact of attachment disturbances or significant childhood trauma is a necessary—and painful—step towards healing and personal growth. It is important to understand that these experiences can manifest in various ways throughout our lives. As you read through the signs of adult attachment styles below, consider how they may resonate with your own experiences. Additionally, if you are concerned about your own childhood experiences and their potential impact, you might find it helpful to take the Adverse Childhood Experiences (ACE) test.

Adult indications of childhood attachment disorder

Insecure adult attachment styles arise when childhood attachment disorder remains unresolved. It is a continuation of the self-protective behaviors that first emerged in childhood, but which now affect a person's adult relationships. These attachment styles—anxious, avoidant, and fearful-avoidant (disorganized)—can deeply influence how we form relationships.

Anxious attachment: Individuals with anxious attachment may find themselves preoccupied with fears of abandonment or rejection. This often leads to hypersensitivity and overreactions, manifesting in behaviors such as catastrophic thinking, explosive anger in the face of perceived threats, and difficulty handling criticism. Despite viewing others positively, they may struggle with a negative self-image and go to great lengths to maintain relationships through pleasing behaviors often at the expense of their own needs.

Avoidant attachment: Those with avoidant attachment often fear rejection and intimacy, leading to extreme independence and self-reliance. They may prefer focusing on personal achievements over relationships, and will withdraw from, or sabotage, relationships requiring increased intimacy. People with this attachment style may repress or deny their strong feelings, have difficulty accepting help or seeking support, and often have a high level of distrust for others since they have the expectation of rejection. An outward positive self-regard may often compensate for low self-worth.

Fearful-avoidant (disorganized) attachment: This style combines traits from both anxious and avoidant attachments. Individuals may demonstrate unpredictable behaviors in relationships, alternating between extreme emotional expression and shutting down. While desiring connection and validation, people with this attachment style are simultaneously fearful of connection since it also represents vulnerability and a threat to their safety. They may fluctuate between seeking proximity in relationship one moment, then withdrawing without warning, reflecting a deep struggle with trust and intimacy.

Take the ACE test

Your Adverse Childhood Experiences (ACE) test offers insight into past traumas that may still be affecting you. Each "yes" response to the questions contributes to your ACE score, indicating the number of significant stressors experienced during childhood. As you consider your results, reflect with compassion. This score serves as a tool for understanding rather than a judgment of your worth or potential.

The ACE test can bring about difficult emotions, but it's essential to approach these feelings with self-compassion. Realize that you are not alone and that there are resources and professionals available to help guide and support your healing journey.

Before your 18th birthday:

1. Did a parent or other adult in the household often or very often... a) Swear at you, insult you, put you down, or humiliate you? Or b) Act in a way that made you afraid that you might be physically hurt?

2. Did a parent or other adult in the household often or very often... a) Push, grab, slap, or throw something at you? Or b) Ever hit you so hard that you had marks or were injured?

3. Did an adult or person at least 5 years older than you ever... a) Touch or fondle you or have you touch their body in a sexual way? or b) Attempt or actually have oral, anal, or vaginal intercourse with you?

4. Did you often or very often feel that ... a) No one in your family loved you or thought you were important or special? or b) Your family didn't look out for each other, feel close to each other, or support each other?

5. Did you often or very often feel that ... a) You didn't have enough to eat, had to wear dirty clothes, and had no one to protect you? or b) Your parents were too drunk or high to take care of you or take you to the doctor if you needed it?

6. Were your parents ever separated or divorced?

7. Was your parent/caregiver: a) Often or very often pushed, grabbed, slapped or had something thrown at him/her? or b) Sometimes, often, or very often kicked, bitten, hit with a fist, or hit with something hard? or c) Ever repeatedly hit over at least a few minutes or threatened with a gun or knife?

8. Did you live with anyone who was a problem drinker or alcoholic, or who used street drugs?

9. Was a household member depressed or mentally ill, or did a household member attempt suicide?

10. Did a household member go to prison?

What does your ACE score mean?

Almost two-thirds of adults have at least one ACE and one in every six adults has a score of 4 or greater.[9,10]

0-3 points: A lower score typically indicates that you have experienced fewer adversities in childhood. While this is a positive outcome, it is still essential to acknowledge that everyone faces challenges, and experiences can vary widely.

4-6 points: A moderate score indicates a higher likelihood of experiencing emotional, psychological and physical health challenges later in life. This score suggests that you may be at an increased risk for various health issues, including anxiety, depression, and chronic illnesses. Recognizing this can empower you to seek support and make proactive choices about your well-being.

7 points or higher: A higher score correlates with a significantly increased risk for various health and emotional challenges. Individuals with these scores may experience profound effects on their mental and physical health. Understanding this connection can be a crucial step toward seeking help, building resilience, and implementing strategies for healing.

Post-traumatic growth: Adversity is opportunity

Bringing these insights together can be an enlightening, albeit challenging, process. If you find that you relate to any attachment concerns or have an ACE score reflecting significant childhood trauma, seeking support from a trained therapist can be incredibly beneficial. Healing often happens through relationships, whether with yourself, others, or the broader world. Recognizing how early experiences shape your adult life is a courageous step in your pursuit of well-being. Embrace the journey toward healing with openness and compassion, understanding that real growth is always possible.

Post-traumatic growth (PTG) refers to the positive psychological transformations that can occur following a traumatic event. This concept, extensively researched by psychologists Richard Tedeschi and Lawrence Calhoun, provides hope that beyond mere recovery to baseline, trauma survivors can achieve profound personal growth.[11] Tedeschi and Calhoun's research is well validated; one review of PTG studies showed that 30 to 70 percent of individuals who survive various traumatic events report positive changes in their lives as a result.[12]

What is essential to keep in mind is that PTG is not a direct result of the trauma itself, but instead related to how the individual struggles as a result of the trauma.[13,14]

For individuals with GERD, navigating its emotional and psychological challenges, along with the challenge of its chronic physical symptoms can similarly lead to transformative growth. A true understanding of GERD necessitates a deep dive into our emotional landscape where we can begin to pull apart the craggy rocks of experience in order to find meaning. This is the same meaning that Tedeschi and Calhoun allude to while seeking to explain the phenomenon of post-traumatic growth.

Managing our triggers

When past traumas do resurface, they can sometimes manifest as overwhelming triggers that make us feel unsafe and disoriented. It is crucial to have tools at our disposal to help navigate these challenging moments. Grounding and centering exercises are practical strategies designed to anchor us in the present, providing a sense of stability and security when faced with distress. These techniques can interrupt cycles of anxiety and help us reconnect with a feeling of safety, both physically and emotionally. As you explore the following exercises, consider how they might be integrated into your daily routine as ongoing resources for managing trauma-related stress and promoting overall well-being.

Exercise 20.1: Grounding into the present

Grounding is a powerful technique that helps to set aside our intrusive feelings, thoughts, and memories of the past, allowing us to reconnect with the present moment. Follow these steps whenever you need a reminder of your safety, resilience, and tranquility.

1. **Affirm your safety:** Begin by affirming your current safety. Silently or aloud, tell yourself, "I am safe now." Acknowledge that, regardless of past experiences, you are better equipped to handle any memories that may arise.

2. **Acknowledge your resources:** Remind yourself of the resources that you have to cope with challenges. Repeat affirmations such as, "I have the strength and resilience to face whatever comes my way."

3. **Focus on your breath:** Take a moment to focus on your breathing. Inhale deeply through your nose, allowing your breath to fill your abdomen. Exhale slowly through your mouth. As you breathe in, visualize inhaling calmness, and as you breathe out, let go of tension or stress.

4. **Connect with your body:** Bring awareness to your body as an anchor to the present. Notice your feet planted firmly on the floor. Feel the weight of your body pressing into the ground. Visualize this connection growing stronger as you imagine your awareness moving closer to Earth's center. Take a moment to savor this feeling of support.

5. **Find a comfort object:** If you need tangible comfort, hold an object with special meaning to you. As you breathe in calmness, allow this object to ground you further.

6. **State your age and the date:** To reinforce your presence in this moment, state aloud your age and today's date. This simple act helps to anchor you in the present reality.

7. **Expand your awareness of the environment:** Take a few moments to observe your surroundings. Notice the sights,

sounds, and smells in your environment. Pay attention to the clouds drifting in the sky, the gentle rustle of the wind through the trees, or the warmth of the sun on your skin. Engage your senses with details like the texture of your sofa, the aroma of fresh coffee, or the page number of an open book nearby.

8. **Completion:** Take a final deep breath and know that you are capable of thriving, and when challenges arise, you can always return to this practice for safety and peace.

Exercise 20.2: Peaceful in the center

This centering exercise invites you to create a personal sanctuary of peace within your imagination, harnessing the power of visualization to cultivate feelings of tranquility and revitalization.

1. **Create your personal image library:** Begin by gathering images that represent peace, tranquility, and revitalization for you. These could be photographs, drawings, or even descriptions of places that evoke a sense of calm. Take a few moments to reflect on what these images mean to you and how they make you feel.

2. **Connect with each image:** Focus on each image in turn. Allow yourself to fully engage with the visuals, immersing yourself in the feelings they evoke. Ask yourself: What emotions come up? Where do I feel this in my body?

3. **Visualize your personal sanctuary:** Now, close your eyes and imagine that the peaceful feelings you have cultivated are physically present in the space around your heart. Visualize a sanctuary that embodies these elements of peace.

- What colors dominate your sanctuary? Are they soft pastels, vibrant greens, or calm blues?

- What sounds fill the air? Perhaps the gentle rustling of leaves, the soothing sound of water, or soft music?

- What fragrances permeate your space? The scent of herbs, fresh earth, or a hint of the ocean?

- Who is with you in your sanctuary? If you prefer solitude, visualize the natural elements that populate your space—the flowers, trees, or animals that add life to your tranquil haven.

4. **Engage your senses:** Pay attention to the sensations around you. What do you feel on your skin? Is it the sun's warmth, a gentle breeze, or the coolness of a shaded area?

5. **Breathe in gratitude:** With each in-breath, inhale the gratitude you feel for your sanctuary. Let this feeling fill your entire being, appreciating the revitalizing effects it has on you. While exhaling, notice how your presence in this sanctuary completes the space. Visualize it responding to you as if recognizing your need for peace and connection.

6. **Allow the connection to grow:** Take a few moments to let the feelings of connection flourish. Allow this visualization to shift and change as needed, making it uniquely yours.

7. **Gradually return:** When you feel ready, gently bring your awareness back to your physical surroundings. Open your eyes, and take a moment to reflect on the experience. Consider journaling any insights or feelings that arose during the exercise.

By regularly practicing this centering exercise, you can cultivate a sanctuary of peace within yourself that you can return to whenever you need a moment of calm and connection.

Unbounded connection

We are always and in every way seeking connection. We each demonstrate different behaviors through which to connect with others, but feelings are fundamental to all our efforts at connection. Healing involves identifying and working with our negative feeling states, which are reflected back at us whether in relationship with self, another, nature, or a higher power.

If you have a predominantly negative feeling state or you display signs of unresolved trauma, this is your cue to seek help. Our past experiences are encoded into our negative feelings and need not define or limit us. Enormous personal growth is possible when we pay attention to those aspects of our life that cause us the greatest discomfort.

---

1. Cochrane, A. L., Cochrane, A., & Blythe, M., (1989). One man's medicine: An autobiography of Professor Archie Cochrane. London, UK; British Medical Journal.

2. Goldberg, S., Muir, R., & Kerr, J., (eds.), (1995). Attachment theory: Social, developmental, and clinical perspectives. Hillsdale, NJ, USA; The Analytic Press, Inc.

3. Ross, T., & Pfäfflin, F., (2007). Attachment and interpersonal problems in a prison environment. *Journal of Forensic Psychiatry and Psychology*, 18(1): 90-98.

4. Langton, C.M., Murad, Z., & Humbert, B., (2017). Childhood sexual abuse, attachments in childhood and adulthood, and coercive sexual behaviors in community males. *Sexual Abuse*, 29(3): 207-238.

5. Levy, T.M., & Orleans, M., (2014). Attachment, trauma, and healing: Understanding and treating attachment disorder in children, families and adults. Philadelphia, PA, USA; Jessica Kingsley Publishers.

6. Smallbone, S.W., & Dadds, M.R., (2000). Attachment and coercive sexual behavior. *Sexual Abuse*, 12(1): 3-15.

7. Pat-Horenczyk, R., Brom, D., & Vogel, J.M., (eds.), (2014). Helping children cope with trauma: Individual, family and community perspectives. New York, NY, USA; Routledge.

8. Hornor, G., (2019). Attachment disorders. *Journal of Pediatric Health Care,* 33(5): 612-622.

9. Felitti, V. J., Anda, R. F., Nordenberg, D., Williamson, D. F., Spitz, A. M., Edwards, V., Koss, M. P., & Marks, J. S., (1998). Relationship of childhood abuse and household dysfunction to many of the leading causes of death in adults. The Adverse Childhood Experiences (ACE) Study. *American Journal of Preventive Medicine,* 14(4): 245-258.

10. Dong, M., Anda, R. F., Felitti, V. J., Dube, S. R., Williamson, D. F., Thompson, T. J., Loo, C. M., & Giles, W. H., (2004). The interrelatedness of multiple forms of childhood abuse, neglect, and household dysfunction. *Child Abuse & Neglect,* 28(7): 771-784.

11. Tedeschi, R. G., & Calhoun, L. G., (1996). The Posttraumatic Growth Inventory: Measuring the positive legacy of trauma. *Journal of Traumatic Stress,* 9(3): 455-471.

12. Linley, P. A., & Joseph, S., (2004). Positive change following trauma and adversity: A review. *Journal of Traumatic Stress,* 17(1): 11-21.

13. Tedeschi, R. G., & Calhoun, L. G., (2004). Posttraumatic growth: Conceptual foundation and empirical evidence. *Psychological Inquiry,* 15(1): 1-18.

14. Calhoun, L. G., & Tedeschi, R. G., (2004). The foundations of posttraumatic growth: New considerations. *Psychological Inquiry,* 15(1): 93-102.

Part IV: Generative Healing

*"The mystery of life is not a problem to be solved;
it is reality to be experienced."*

— Johannes Jacobus van der Leeuw, The Conquest of Illusion

TWENTY-ONE

Self-Nurturing: Ideas for Filling Your Bucket

Unlocking the abundance of your inner landscape

On our journey of self-awareness and enhanced well-being, there are always opportunities for profound personal growth. One such opportunity is in our innate capacity for generativity—the ways in which we create, vitalize, nurture and contribute meaningfully to the world around us. Generativity represents our commitment and connections to others in ways that are wholly realized only when we first nurture ourselves.

We can think of our bucket as a rich inner reservoir to be filled with the self-nourishing resources we uncover along our journeys. Just as miners sift through the earth in search of precious gold and gemstones, we too can excavate our beautiful and deep treasures and—through constant reminder, rediscovery, and renewed insight—we fill our buckets with our personal gems.

This chapter will guide you through practical exercises to help you tap into these hidden treasures. The focus here is on enhancing your emotional well-being and resilience by connecting with the positive aspects of your experiences. By centering your exploration on generativity, you can shift the narrative from one of suppression, repression, and depression to a more fulfilling and empowering mindset. As you engage with these exercises, approach them with an open heart and a curious mind. Allow yourself to explore and nurture the feelings that arise, recognizing that each step you take contributes to filling your inner reservoir—your bucket.

Exercise 21.1: What I like to do

Take a moment to reflect on and list all the activities that bring you joy and fulfillment. For each activity, write down specific aspects that make it enjoyable, how it makes you feel, and why it resonates with you. Use the template below to guide your thoughts.

My list of favorite activities

Activity: _____
What I like about it: _____
How it makes me feel: _____
Why it resonates with me: _____

Examples

Activity: Skiing
What I like about it: It's an activity I've shared with my favorite people of all time.
How it makes me feel: It gets me in a space of flow where everything just feels so effortless.
Why it resonates with me: It brings out my joie de vivre.

Activity: Reading nonfiction
What I like about it: I love diving into new ideas and real-life accounts that provide insights for personal growth.
How it makes me feel: It sparks my imagination and enriches my understanding of the possibilities for the world, while prompting me to think critically about various topics.
Why it resonates with me: Reading nonfiction allows me to gain knowledge and appreciate diverse perspectives, fostering empathy

in my life by connecting me to the diverse experiences and stories of others.

Once you have finished your list, consider how each activity helps you connect with yourself, others, the planet, or your higher power. Make this list as extensive as possible, exploring everything that energizes you and makes you feel alive and grounded, no matter what is happening in your life. Refer to your list often, adding new activities as you discover them. Use this resource to shift from negative feelings to a more positive state. Then, choose an activity that resonates with you and make time to engage in it. Remember, you deserve to engage in the things that uplift and nourish you!

Exercise 21.2: My best memories

Take a moment to reflect on and list your favorite memories, including all the elements that contributed to those good moments in your life. Consider the people, places, events, senses, and feelings that made these experiences special. Use the template below to guide your thoughts.

My list of best memories

Memory: _____
People involved: _____
Places: _____
Events: _____
Senses: _____
Feelings: _____
Why it's special: _____

Examples

Memory: My wedding day.
People involved: My wife, family, friends.
Places: The stunning natural beauty and enchanting scenes of the wedding venue.
Events: The ceremony, reception, and celebration.
Senses: The sound of laughter, the scent of wild thyme, the feel of my wife's hand in mine.
Feelings: Joy, love, gratitude.
Why it's special: This day marked the beginning of our married life together, surrounded by loved ones who shared in our happiness with the warmth of their support.

Memory: Climbing a mountain by day and exiting its forest shroud into the mountain valley at night.
People involved: My friend and I.
Places: The braided river, mountain valley, and surrounding mountain ranges.
Events: The climb, the nighttime descent into the mountain valley, and witnessing a sky full of stars.
Senses: The crisp mountain air, the sound of rustling leaves, the sight of the expansive sky, and the chill of the night breeze.
Feelings: Awe, exhilaration, peace.
Why it's special: This experience was a profound connection to nature, where the transition from day to night symbolized the beauty of life's journey, culminating in the breathtaking view of the stars and the magical moment of seeing a shooting star.

Once you have completed your list, reference it regularly to remind yourself of the beautiful moments in your own life. Remembering good times is a powerful way to build resilience, especially when negative thoughts and anticipations creep in. This exercise not only helps you cherish your joyful memories, but also serves as a reminder of the richness of your experiences, some of which you may have forgotten over time. Take this opportunity to explore your best memories and allow them to uplift and inspire you. Fill your life with recollections that fuel your resilience and joy!

Exercise 21.3: My strengths and achievements

Take a moment to reflect on and list all your achievements, no matter how big or small, from as far back as you can remember. Consider your strengths, including those recognized by others through feedback or compliments. This is a personal exercise focused on celebrating you, so embrace the opportunity to acknowledge everything you are proud of. Use the template below to guide your thoughts.

My list of strengths and achievements

Achievement: _____
Strength/skill: _____
Date/time period: _____
Feelings about achievement: _____
Why it's important to me: _____

Examples

Achievement: Choosing to prioritize life by not taking my own at age 16.
Strength/skill: Resilience and courage.
Date/time period: 1987.
Feelings about achievement: Grateful, relieved, and empowered.
Why it's important to me: This choice was a pivotal moment in my life, marking the beginning of a lifelong commitment toward

healing and self-acceptance. It showed me that I have the strength to overcome hardship, and it established a foundation of resilience for the extraordinary highs and lows that followed. Reflecting on this moment helps me to appreciate that I am at my most real when I can acknowledge my shadow, and to be open with others and seek help when needed.

Achievement: Learning to build houses for the first time following a mid-life turning point.
Strength/skill: Adaptability and determination.
Date/time period: Since 2023.
Feelings about achievement: Excited, accomplished, and proud.
Why it's important to me: This experience opened up new possibilities for me and allowed me to connect my hands with my head while serving others. It reinforces my belief that it is never too late to learn something new and make a meaningful impact in my community. Being able to create something tangible gives me a sense of purpose and connection to others and highlights the resilience of the human spirit.

If creating your list is a struggle, remember that simply getting out of bed each day is an achievement. This can be especially true during low mood when positive self-regard becomes challenging. You might also consider creating a side list of qualities that you appreciate in others, which can serve as a reminder of your own worth. If you see goodness in others, it is a reflection of the good that exists within you too. Once you have completed your primary list, refer to it often, adding new accomplishments and strengths as you become more aware of your positive attributes. Over time, this exercise can help you cultivate a deeper appreciation for your journey and the unique strengths that you bring to the world.

Exercise 21.4: Things I hope to do

Take a moment to reflect on all the things you hope to do and achieve—your personal bucket list. Allow your imagination to run wild and don't hesitate to think big; be outrageous if you need to! As you write each aspiration, include the feelings you anticipate experiencing as you pursue these goals. Use the template below to guide your thoughts.

My bucket list: Aspirations and hopes

I hope to: _____
Feelings I will experience: _____

I hope to: _____
Feelings I will experience: _____

If you find it challenging to create a bucket list due to low mood or other barriers, consider an alternative approach by writing affirmations about your future. This can help cultivate a positive mindset and reinforce your belief in your potential. Here are some examples for inspiration:

- I choose a good life filled with joy and purpose.

- I deserve to feel loved and appreciated in my relationships.

- I plan to make my life count by pursuing my passions.

- I am getting stronger every day, overcoming obstacles along the way.

- I hope to enjoy the company of my grandchildren and create lasting memories.

- I intend to live fully, embracing gratitude and mindfulness.

- I have much to offer, and am excited to develop my potential further.

- I have had experiences of value that I can share with others to inspire and uplift them.

- I plan to travel and explore new cultures, enriching my understanding of the world.

- I aim to strengthen my relationships with everyone in my life, cultivating deeper connections.

Once you have completed your list of affirmations, revisit them regularly to remind yourself of your hopes and dreams. Embrace the possibility of these becoming a reality, and allow this exercise to energize and motivate you as you move forward in life!

Heart coherence and the "Heart Lock-in" technique

As you continue to reflect on your goldmine and the ways in which you add value—not only to yourself, but also the world—it is important to consider ways to elevate your baseline emotional state to facilitate achieving these goals. One powerful way to do this is by harnessing the concept of heart coherence, which allows us to perform at our highest potential in whatever we choose to pursue. Most people are familiar with the idea of "peak experiences"—those blissful moments when we find ourselves "in the flow," where everything seems effortless, and we feel a deep connection with those around us.

High-performance athletes often rely on such experiences to push their limits and achieve greater success. Many individuals report experiencing these peaks during moments of stillness, such as fasting or prayer, as well as when engaging in music, art, or other creative endeavors. The beauty is that we all possess the capacity to tap into these enriching moments of coherence.

Heart coherence is a physiologically measurable state, demonstrating that our heart can be a powerful tool for intentional change. One important measurement of this coherence is heart rate variability (HRV), which we first looked at in *GERD—the dualistic biomedical perspective*. HRV refers to the natural beat-to-beat variation in heart rate. When a person is in a coherent state, their heart exhibits high beat-to-beat variation (high HRV). In contrast, states of frustration or stress typically yield low HRV.

This distinction is important because low HRV correlates with stress and the shutting down of the brain's frontal cortex, which is responsible for learning and problem-solving. Instead, our neurological focus is diverted to the hindbrain, preparing for fight, flight, or freeze responses. In individuals facing serious health challenges, such as GERD or advanced cancer, low HRV has been associated with worsening health outcomes. Conversely, when a person is in a coherent state (high HRV), the heart communicates vital messages to the frontal cortex, making it primed for learning, creativity, and effective decision-making. High HRV is associated with better test performance, enhanced problem-solving abilities, and improved health outcomes.[1,2,3]

Somehow, when we are in a coherent state, colors just seem richer, food tastes better, and the world is more vibrant, accepting and peaceful.

Exercise 21.5: The "Heart Lock-in" technique

The Heart Lock-in technique is a simple 3-step procedure that you can use to shift from low HRV to a coherent, high HRV state. It can be learned in a few minutes and is easily made a part of your daily, intentional well-being practice. Scientists at the nonprofit Institute of HeartMath (IHM)[4] have shown that practicing this simple technique for just five minutes a day can significantly benefit your overall well-being.[5] Here's how to do it:

1. **Heart awareness:** Create awareness of the space around your heart.

2. **Heart breathing:** Breathe as if you are breathing into and

out of your heart, paying attention to your breath and noticing how it becomes slower and deeper.

3. **Heart appreciation:** Think of someone or something that you feel a genuine sense of appreciation, compassion, or gratitude toward; while holding this feeling, continue breathing into and out of your heart, noticing the sense of aliveness that arises from within.

---

1. Bradley, R.T., McCraty, R., Atkinson, M., Tomasino, D., Daugherty, A., & Arguelles, L., (2010). Emotion self-regulation, psychophysiological coherence, and test anxiety: results from an experiment using electrophysiological measures. *Applied Psychophysiology and Biofeedback,* 35(4): 261-283.

2. McCraty, R., & Atkinson, M., (2012). Resilience training program reduces physiological and psychological stress in police officers. *Global Advances in Health and Medicine,* 1(5): 44-66.

3. McCraty, R., (2022). Following the rhythm of the heart: HeartMath Institute's path to HRV biofeedback. *Applied Psychophysiology and Biofeedback,* 47(4): 305-316.

4. www.heartmath.org

5. McCraty, R., Barrios-Choplin, B., Rozman, D., Atkinson, M., & Watkins, A. D., (1998). The impact of a new emotional self-management program on stress, emotions, heart rate variability, DHEA and cortisol. *Integrative Pscyhological and Behavioral Science,* 33(2): 151-170.

TWENTY-TWO

Getting Therapeutic Support for GERD

A natural fit for a meaning-based story approach

When I speak of therapeutic support, I acknowledge my own experiences and preferences, which lean toward psychotherapeutic, counseling or "talk therapy" approaches. I have not had a lot of experience with body-focused healing modalities—outside many informative experiences with biomedicine—but willingly acknowledge that these modalities have a place in the postmodern therapeutic space.

So while this chapter focuses on talk therapy, other modalities such as Complementary and Alternative Medicine (CAM) can also be valuable.[1] A therapeutic massage, for example, can be helpful for exploring and expressing difficult body sensations. A massage practitioner who understands the story behind these symptoms and encourages you to safely explore that narrative is invaluable to your experience.

I personally see talk therapy as a natural "fit" for a meaning-based story approach and envision a future in which all practitioners are trained in a MindBody or wholeperson approach to facilitate healing of chronic "physical" diseases, while using the same methods to become more proficient in healing "psychological" wounding. In this progression, I see the postmodern therapist as increasingly *less* differentiated from the ancient shaman.

Indeed, I firmly reject any attempt to separate disease or suffering of any kind into compartments of convenience that subsequently dictate scope of practice. Once a person's emergent and acute needs have been addressed through biomedicine, my view is that an empathetic, *deep*-listening and well-supervised MindBody practitioner is more suited to helping a person with triple-positive stage III breast cancer, NYHA class III heart failure or treatment-refractory GERD than an oncologist, cardiologist or gastroenterologist. When a person's "physical" illness has progressed to these stages despite state-of-the-art care from allopathic medicine, surely this is an admission that a meaning-based story approach holds validity?

"Insanity is doing the same thing over and over again and expecting different results."

— Rita Mae Brown, civil rights campaigner

A word of caution: Caveat emptor

I have experienced therapy with traditional talk therapists who have not yet developed the necessary nuances in their psychodynamic or depth psychology practices to effectively address the types of issues that clients ordinarily bring to them. Such therapists would struggle to make any positive impact for a client who comes to them for help with their GERD.

Some therapists—due to their training with the biomedical model—may prioritize pathologizing a person's symptoms and behaviors over a more relational approach geared toward wholeperson healing. I personally have had terrible experiences with practitioners trained in clinical psychology; they lacked empathy and over-emphasized the use of cognitive-behavioral therapy (CBT) or one of its subtle but shallow variants. CBT focuses on a person's observable and measurable signs at the exclusion of our individual subjectivity.[2]

The field of "dualistic psychology" is as troubled as medicine. Clinical psychology largely defines this area, having evolved as a complementary paradigm to medicine. Both focus on evidence-based therapies and practices at the expense of a person's subjective story. It is crucial to recognize that much of the dysfunction in medicine and clinical psychology stems from allied industries that prioritize their own interests, funding studies to "supply" evidence that benefits it. As we know from our experiences of GERD, the medicalization of our symptoms only leads to the persistence of symptoms. The medicalization of the mind is similarly troubling and explains why many "mind" practitioners leave their clients feeling misunderstood or unheard, as their problems are reduced to a set of behaviors.

None of this means that one type of practitioner is better than another. Despite the crisis of dualism and its evidence-based conundrum, I believe we can be somewhat assured that:

- Postmodern training programs across clinical as well as traditional psychotherapeutic disciplines are now focused on integrating relational and contextual approaches to achieve person-centered care.

- In some territories, the use of CBT and its variants is becoming more nuanced in order to include client narratives and relationships, alongside the cognitive work that resembles the reframes we discussed in *Accepting and reframing feelings through energy psychology*.

- Through continuing education programs, practitioners around the world are encouraged to explore and deepen their practice philosophies that underlie all assumptions about the wholeperson.

"MindBody" and "Mind—Body" are not the same

For your GERD, I recommend finding a therapist who has a MindBody or wholeperson understanding of disease and its underlying personal story.

Be a little wary of therapists who refer to "integrative approaches," "the mind–body connection," "Mind–Body," or in some other way imply that mind and body are separate. Used in this way, these are mere buzz words to imply cognizance of the role of emotions in our physical symptoms. All the while, the unenlightened practitioner ignores the underlying MindBody philosophy that recognizes emotions, stories and symptoms as fundamentally the same thing. The result can be a practice that is just as hyphenated as the words used to describe it. Even the term "MindBody" implies there is separation between mind and body by virtue of the different names given to the component domains.

At this juncture, only a small minority of talk therapists may recognize that GERD is not simply a physical condition but one that necessitates a wholeperson perspective for its effective resolution. I sincerely hope change comes soon. Your willingness to embrace these ideas is crucial for this change.

For this reason, you need to be careful who you choose to support you. And having found someone, you might just need to lead them on a journey of their own! Your continued progress will be difficult if your therapist has doubts about the importance of story in *every* illness, including your GERD.

The trick as far as you are concerned is seeing beyond the therapist's label, title and credentials in order to learn about what they really offer and whether this aligns with your needs. Even then you will only know if your therapist is a good fit once you have a session or two together. Finding the right therapist is not as random as kissing frogs, but there are some useful things to keep in mind to make a suitable match.

Reasons for seeking support

The remainder of this chapter is specifically intended for you if:

- Your physical GERD symptoms have improved or resolved, but you feel that unresolved emotional issues remain; or,

- You have had limited success resolving GERD symptoms independently and want therapeutic support; or,

- You need guidance on finding a suitable therapist.

> **IMPORTANT:** Please seek immediate professional help if you experience thoughts of self-harm, hallucinations, or you feel you are losing touch with reality.

Possible issues that you may be struggling with, and which you can expect to receive help for include:

- I want to gain awareness of my embodied feelings and GERD triggers.
- I want to learn to accept difficult feelings and thoughts.
- I want to develop healthier ways to express my feelings and improve self-esteem.
- I want to prioritize my self-care while honoring the ways I previously coped with trauma and loss.
- I want to overcome maladaptive thoughts and behaviors.
- I want to increase my self-awareness and relationship skills.
- I want to adequately grieve past losses.
- I want to process and release strong negative feelings.
- I want to feel more appreciative of myself, others, and my community.
- I want to identify my strengths, gifts, and purpose.
- I want to find inner peace.

Preparing for therapy

Before approaching prospective therapists, your preparation may include a personal stock take of your present resources (see: *Self-nurturing: Ideas for filling your bucket*.) Therapy is a commitment so you need to have the emotional and practical resources in place to sustain you along your journey.

Your immediate safety needs are paramount, and certainly take priority over beginning therapy. When you are feeling safe from harm and your basic daily needs are met, then it may be time to think about starting therapy. Questions you can ask yourself to determine your readiness include: Am I safe? Do I have my food and shelter needs met? Do I have the minimum practical resources and life balance to sustain me?

Seeking out a therapist when someone pressures you into going is never a good idea. That is not to say you should not consider therapy if someone raises the idea with you. But there should never be pressure involved. As long as you have your own reasons for going and you welcome having support to make changes in your life that you want to make, then therapy is likely right for you.

Some people are ready for therapy but fail to take the final leap due to finding obstacles constantly in their path. If this sounds like you, it is worthwhile practicing a little mindfulness next time an obstacle appears. Focus on the obstacle as a detached but curious observer rather than as someone caught up in its drama. Then ask yourself if the obstacle in question warrants you abandoning your own need for personal growth. Sometimes we just need to take the final leap, no matter what.

Cost and access concerns

United States

Access to talk therapy in the U.S. is highly dependent on insurance coverage, with private policies often dictating terms such as number of therapy sessions per year, types of therapies covered, and pre-authorization requirements. High deductibles and copayments can be significant barriers, alongside limited sessions and the challenge of finding in-network providers to keep out-of-pocket expenses low. Even if therapy is covered, high copays can make the commitment to care financially burdensome. While the Affordable Care Act improved coverage for mental health, disparities persist. Private funding gaps and administrative hurdles often act as gatekeepers, restricting timely access to services. Clients may additionally worry about privacy, as insurance claims require sharing personal information.

Canada

Canada offers a mix of public and private funding for mental health services. While provincial health plans provide some coverage, talk therapy with a psychologist or counselor typically requires private insurance or out-of-pocket payment. Accessibility can vary widely depending on personal or employer-provided insurance and the availability of mental health professionals.

Europe

Access to talk therapy in Europe varies by country but generally features a stronger public health component. Many European nations have national healthcare systems that offer broad mental health coverage; however, wait times can pose challenges. In countries with dual public-private systems, like Germany and France, private insurance can enhance access but may also create disparities based on socioeconomic status.

United Kingdom

In the UK, the National Health Service (NHS) provides access to mental health services, including talk therapy. The main barrier is often long wait times due to high demand and limited resources. Private therapy is available but can be costly. The focus on expanding community-based mental health programs is helping improve accessibility over time.

Australia

Australia's public healthcare system, Medicare, offers some subsidized sessions with psychologists under the Mental Health Treatment Plan, though there are limits on the number of subsidized sessions. Additional sessions require out-of-pocket payment or private insurance, which can hinder access for some. The Better Access initiative aims to improve accessibility, but geographical disparities exist, affecting those in rural or remote areas more severely.

New Zealand

New Zealand provides mental health services through its public healthcare system, but access can be uneven. While government funding covers some mental health services, including emergency and community support, wait times can be long. Private therapy can be expensive, creating a financial barrier for those without insurance or adequate coverage from primary health organizations.

The common threads affecting access to talk therapy include the balance between public and private funding, the extent and nature of insurance coverage, and logistical factors like wait times and availability of professionals. These elements collectively influence how easily individuals can access mental health support, with financial resources often serving as a key determinant.

Enhancing access to essential care

If access is a personal concern for you, there are several emergent trends aimed at enhancing access to talk therapy. Notable developments include tele-therapy and online counseling, which have gained significant traction post-pandemic. Online therapy services have started to facilitate cross-border access to care, allowing individuals to connect with therapists in different territories when local options are limited and cost of care is prohibitive.

Many healthcare systems are increasingly integrating mental health services with primary care. This model allows patients to receive psychological support alongside physical health services, and may in future become the main point of care for MindBody or wholeperson approaches. In many regions, there has been a notable increase in public health awareness campaigns highlighting the importance of mental health and the availability of resources, and directing individuals toward support. Policymakers in some territories are working toward mental health insurance reform, aiming to ensure that therapy is treated with the same importance as physical health.

Finally, the rise of mental health apps is facilitating broader access to therapeutic resources, including mindfulness exercises and other self-help tools.

While these do not replace traditional talk therapy, they can provide individuals with immediate support and augment their healing journey. As mental health continues to be prioritized globally, we can expect further innovations to enhance availability of care.

Beyond labels: Therapy's different forms and flavors

The terms "counselor" and "psychotherapist" are interchangeable in most countries, yet the variances in terminology reflect the diverse approaches available to those seeking support. While counselor is a modern term frequently employed in territories where psychotherapist is a protected title, it also serves as an important way to destigmatize the therapeutic journey. Both titles represent professionals dedicated to the practice of soul healing, which is the literal meaning of psychotherapy. Importantly, the distinction between these titles does not imply differences in training or qualifications; someone identifying as a counselor can possess the same expertise and capabilities as a psychotherapist.

When searching for a therapist, the term "psychologist" often comes up. This is such a broad term with academic, industry and clinical implications, and may not be especially helpful in finding a therapist with a particular set of listening and empathy skills appropriate for healing relationships.

Today, the integration of various philosophies—gestalt, existentialist, humanistic, cognitive-behavioral, feminist, systems, postmodern, and Mind-Body—has enriched therapeutic practice and created a spectrum of care models to suit everyone's unique needs. Therapy welcomes individuals from all backgrounds, both as practitioners and clients, highlighting that effective support comes in many flavors.

Training programs across universities and specialized institutes ensure that aspiring therapists are exposed to a rich variety of philosophies and receive robust supervision as they prepare and continue to engage with their clients. This diversity within the field reflects the idea that there is no one-size-fits-all approach to healing, encouraging everyone to explore the therapeutic avenue that resonates most with them.

Therapeutic frames

A narrow view

The therapeutic frame in psychotherapy is perhaps the most important concept to grasp when considering your therapeutic journey. In its narrowest sense, the frame encompasses the various fixed elements that are always in place whenever you and your therapist meet—whether virtually, in-person, one-on-one, in groups, or through prepared programs. In addition to the setting, the frame defines the length and frequency of sessions, therapeutic goals, and professional ethics. Regardless of the shape it takes, the frame establishes the boundaries for the work that you will do together with your therapist, including limits on personal disclosure and any rules regarding contact outside the session.

Virtual (online) therapy: Virtual therapy has gained immense popularity, offering convenience and flexibility to attend sessions from the comfort of your home. Through secure video conferencing platforms, you can engage in real-time conversations with your therapist, making it a practical option for those with busy schedules or mobility challenges. However, there are downsides; therapists may struggle to pick up on nonverbal cues like body language, which can provide important insights into a client's feelings. Some therapists find that virtual meetings lack the intimacy of in-person encounters, and may impact their understanding of transference (the feelings clients project onto their therapist) and countertransference (the therapist's emotional responses to the client), potentially complicating the therapeutic relationship.

In-person one-on-one therapy: Traditional in-person therapy remains a choice for many people. Some people find that meeting face-to-face allows for a deeper emotional connection, as body language, eye contact, and physical presence play crucial roles in communication. This format fosters a sense of accountability and can create a safe space for honest exploration of your feelings. However, some individuals may feel intimidated or vulnerable in this setting, which could hinder their ability to open up. The physical environment can also be a double-edged sword; while it can offer stability, it may also evoke anxiety for some.

In-person group therapy: Group therapy provides a unique opportunity to share experiences and learn from others under the guidance of a trained facilitator. This format can foster a sense of belonging and reduce feelings of isolation. Participants often find strength in knowing that they are not alone in their struggles. However, group settings can also feel overwhelming or intimidating for some individuals, making it difficult to share personal challenges. Additionally, the dynamics of the group may lead to competing voices that can overshadow individual experiences.

Prepared programs: Workshops and structured group therapy focus on specific themes such as trauma recovery or stress management. They offer participants practical tools and strategies for addressing challenges. These programs can create a supportive atmosphere while also facilitating connections among individuals with similar goals. On the downside, some clients may feel that a structured program limits personal attention compared to one-on-one therapy, which can be crucial for more nuanced emotional exploration.

Hybrid therapy: A hybrid approach combines both in-person and virtual therapy, providing the flexibility to meet clients' needs. This model allows for in-person sessions when possible, along with virtual options when schedules or circumstances dictate. While this can be an effective way to maintain continuity of care, it may also create inconsistencies in the therapeutic relationship. For example, switching between formats can lead to misunderstandings around emotional cues, making it harder for both clients and therapists to navigate transference and countertransference.

Each of these meeting formats has its unique strengths and weaknesses. It is important for individuals to consider what resonates with them and aligns with their own needs. Finding the right approach can significantly enhance the healing journey.

A broad view

In a broader sense, the frame captures the intangible and often unexpressed nuances of the therapeutic space in which you and your therapist relate to one another. It is vital that your therapist invests considerable energy in defining what this space means to them, as it significantly impacts your experience of the relationship. A therapist who has thoughtfully considered this question will likely have sought a firm grounding in their practice philosophy to determine the most effective ways to work with their individual clients.

The boundaries of therapy are more complex than some therapists may acknowledge. By boundaries, I do not just refer to physical elements such as setting, the time of your appointments, fees, cancellations, and whether or not to give your therapist a hug. The boundaries of therapy extend beyond what is explicitly acknowledged in the therapist-client contract to encompass implicit and often unrecognized dimensions.

These implicit aspects of therapeutic boundaries include the following:

- The similarities and differences in how you and your therapist view your suffering.

- Your therapist's willingness to look at suffering from your perspective.

- The openness a therapist has to new information that unexpectedly arises within the therapeutic space (e.g., intuition, gut instincts, etc.).

- Whether the therapist is capable of understanding your suffering through your unique gendered, ethnic, and sociocultural lens.

- The therapist's ability to explore any wider childhood and environmental determinants of your suffering.

- Any limits to the therapist's capacity for empathy and their tolerance for discomfort.

- The theoretical concepts introduced during therapist training and continuing education that may limit or enhance their personal and practice philosophies.

The wholeperson frame

The acknowledgment of a frame in therapy has immediate and practical implications. For example, any therapist who hears you say, "I busted my guts for them," but does not make the possible connection with your GERD is not seeing you as a wholeperson.

Similarly, a therapist who unconsciously suppresses the feeling of nausea they get when you describe an intensely emotional aspect of your story has not learned to see themselves as a wholeperson either. The resonance of our own story in the therapist's body is a boundary of therapy that needs to be explored, whether they are ready to acknowledge it or not. Most practitioners in that situation would unconsciously suppress such a feeling in order to deal with your needs in the present. But in doing so, they would miss the very opportunity your story presented them to have a healing conversation about strong feelings that we experience as nausea.

For this reason, I have included a separate chapter on my website, which you are welcome to share with a prospective talk therapist to open their bodymind and practice to new possibilities. The text is available at https://howardchristian.com/helping-others-a-message-for-talk-therapists/

Consumers of therapy, such as yourself, will drive the positive changes needed for accessible, aspirational and transformational care that places individual, family, community and global well-being as a priority.

Finding the right therapist

Effective therapy, I believe, involves a relational or two-person psychology, which emphasizes the interactions between you and your therapist. It will also contain a psychodynamic component, which allows you and the therapist to bring in any unconscious meanings and motivations. Ideally, your work will be with a therapist who has undergone MindBody or wholeperson training in order to bring in the wholeperson frame described above.

Questions to ask

Review therapist websites for their stated frames and personal philosophies. Don't get bogged down in terminology, but instead focus on the therapist's overall approach. A good therapist, above all, is a great host who prioritizes your needs and is open to your perspectives. Consider scheduling a brief introductory phone call to assess their suitability. Mention upfront your GERD and your desire to approach its healing from a wholeperson perspective. A therapist who lacks this understanding will genuinely believe that they are unable to help you and that is okay. By fronting your issue in this way, you are closer to finding a therapist whose practice philosophies are aligned with your needs.

Use the initial phone call with a therapist as an opportunity to put your instincts to work. Ask yourself, "Is this a person I feel safe and comfortable working with?" Call other therapists to broaden your initial impressions. You do not need to commit to a meeting in person or online just because you made an initial inquiry. Make the final leap only when you are satisfied that there is a good chance the therapist will best serve your needs. If something feels wrong, don't hesitate to seek other options.

Some questions you could ask include:

- What is their training and experience in a MindBody, wholeperson, or meaning-based story approach?
- How long have they been in practice and what are their fees?
- What are their professional affiliations, and code of ethics?
- Do they have experience with online therapy?
- What is their proposed session frequency, and what support do they offer between sessions?

If you are looking at cross-border options for better access to care, it is a good idea to discuss upfront how that would work and what are your rights in the therapist's home territory if you have concerns.

What is important to you?

It is common for people to search for a therapist of the same gender, ethnicity, culture, sexual orientation, or spiritual alignment as themselves. Equally, it is common for people to tolerate and even covet obvious differences between themselves and their prospective therapist.

Either way, there may be conscious and also unconscious reasons for your preference, which may form part of the healthy dynamics and discovery involved in therapy. Some people prioritize the therapist's personality attributes above all else, such as personal warmth, level of engagement, ability to listen, supportiveness, etc. My personal experience is that obvious differences are less important than a therapist's personal attributes. Finding someone who shows you respect and unconditional positive regard is the simplest formula for predicting a transformational therapeutic relationship.

The question of spirituality is subtle. I personally would not choose a therapist who maintains a materialistic worldview, which necessarily excludes common domains of human experience such as belief in a higher power, intuition, interconnectedness of all things, synchronicity and nonlocality, and many other phenomena. But so too would I avoid any therapist who maintains rigid beliefs of a fundamentalist nature, as they are just as likely to harbor unhelpful materialistic assumptions about a separate body and mind.

Your choice of a therapist is essentially based on who will work best for you. This comes with the caveat that a therapist's own assumptions can impact on the progress of your therapy. Look at it this way: If you are on the crest of a transformational moment in your therapy and you hear a door slam or a butterfly flutters through an open window, are you and your therapist attentive to its possible meaning? Only you can answer this. But having your answer, you are a lot closer to finding a therapist who is aligned with your personal growth.

Navigating therapy: The good and the bad

The first therapy session may feel daunting. Remember, it is a step toward meaningful change. Most people feel relief after initial sessions as they begin to process their experiences. This will often involve your therapist finding gentle ways of challenging you. Rather than shying away from these challenges, any accompanying conflict either in yourself or with your therapist is an opportunity for personal discovery.

If your early therapeutic experience feels uncomfortable in another way, reflect on the following list of questions. These are intended to help you assess the direction your therapy is moving and identify any potential issues that may need to be addressed:

1. Does my therapist seem to prioritize my thoughts, thought patterns, and beliefs over my personal story and context related to my struggles?

2. How does my therapist view the role of interpersonal relationships in my experiences? Do they acknowledge how these relationships may contribute to my suffering and healing?

3. Is my therapist open to exploring various therapeutic frameworks, such as psychodynamic, relational, or MindBody approaches, or do they primarily focus on one specific method?

4. Does my therapist emphasize CBT aspects—such as thoughts, behaviors and mood—at the expense of understanding my deeper emotional and relational experiences?

5. How does my therapist handle diagnostic labels? Do they focus excessively on categorizing my suffering rather than understanding my unique experience and personal philosophies that may have developed from early traumas or significant life events?

6. Does my therapist engage in their own personal work or self-reflection to address any significant issues that may affect our therapeutic relationship, or do they seem to operate without this self-awareness?

There is a lot of variety in how prepared a therapist is to show up in a chair across from their client. We are all human after all. But when finding someone to support us may seem like winning the lottery, it is a useful reminder that life is not a problem to be solved, but rather a reality to be experienced. Sometimes we need to have a *bad* experience because this is the standard by which we can know a *good* experience. In life, we attract the people we do because they offer us the lesson we most need to learn at that point in time. I offer this as a personal truth, rather than one of the three laws of thermodynamics.

So, please take a considered approach that reflects your own intuitions and ideas about what you know will work for you.

Changing your mind

If therapy ever feels disrespectful or abusive, back your instincts and respond accordingly. Remember, you can change your mind and look elsewhere for support. Here are some options:

- Discuss your feelings with your therapist.
- If the issue is unresolved, consider speaking to their supervisor.
- If necessary, explore further accountability options—professional bodies, advocacy services—as they apply in your therapist's locale.
- Find a new therapist.

If you ever feel unsafe, leave the session and find a safe place to decide the next steps. Remember, you are the consumer and have rights under your local laws and/or the local laws of the service provider.

A final word

Hopefully your experiences in therapy will be like the majority of people who seek support, with your relationship built around mutual respect and trust. The therapeutic space that your therapist will aim to create with you is intended to allow you to be vulnerable in a safe way, giving you the means to explore any feelings and find personal meaning. You should always feel safe, listened to, viewed with unconditional positive regard, and able to explore your issues in a partnership for your healing.

---

1. CAM, complementary and alternative medicine. The list of body-focused and CAM practices includes: acupuncture; aromatherapy; art therapy; Bowen therapy; breath work therapy; chiropractic; cranio-sacral therapy; EFT; health coaching; homeopathy; iridology; massage therapy; naturopathy; neurolinguistic programing (NLP); osteopathy; pet therapy; podiatry; reflexology; Reiki and other healing touch therapies; shamanic healing, and other traditional healing practices; to name a few.

2. Rowland, H., (2024). Unravelling the dominance: An exploration of the relationship between the medicalisation of ordinary mental distress, the primacy of cognitive behavioural therapy, and the influence of neoliberal ideology in the UK mental health economy. *Medical Research Archives,* 12(5):

Twenty-Three

Why Do We Suffer?

One evening in 2006, during my regular meditation, I experienced a profound spiritual awakening that reshaped my understanding of existence. Variously described as self-realization, transcendence, divine union, nirvikalpa samadhi, satori, non-dual awareness, cosmic or oneness consciousness, and pure subjectivity, this experience required the complete abandonment of ego.

In this moment, the notion of I—the self that clings to embodied identity, personal history, and individual narrative—vanishes into an infinite reality, which the confines of thought and language cannot comprehend.

What unfolds is an expansive realization that consciousness is not limited to human experience, but is instead an essential tapestry of the Whole. As I cease to exist, the Experiencer of this expanded awareness observes an indescribable oneness that transcends all boundaries of form; an immense Stillness. The sensations of body and mind—once felt as a haunting isolation—are cast away, leaving only the pure essence of Being. This essence is not cold, empty or indifferent, but radiates a profound and harmonious warmth—a feeling describable only as love.

In this state of unity, the intricate web of formless existence reveals itself. The Experiencer perceives the Consciousness of all beings—of all things—as flowing from its source. This emergent understanding transforms every concept of individuality and separateness into a mere whisper of illusion. The love I experience transcends mere fleeting emotions; it is the fundamental fabric of All that Is—an unconditional and all-encompassing Love.

The experience obliterates any fear of death, which is realized as a transition—a return to the oneness from which all consciousness emerges. Without our ego's grip, there is nothing to fear losing, for we are always a continuation of the eternal dance of existence. As the Experiencer adjusts the lens of its perception, there is nuance in oneness. I learn that we continue as souls, all sharing the same divine essence while retaining a thread or flavor of discretion whose growth through lifetimes of endeavor serves the continuous expansion and richness of the Whole.

I learn that my suicide now is out of the question since our persistent life-force, the discrete energy signature into which we are co-created, illuminates our karma, soul contracts, and the interconnected journeys we share with one another. A short change in one life demands divine contemplation then repetition in the next until balance is restored.

I realize that our experiences are not random. The lessons we gain especially from suffering are woven into our unique energy signature. Though we may scream our resistance, we ultimately come to understand that we are uniquely predisposed to navigate our own personal trials better than anyone else.

This awakening came with its complexities and challenges. As I strove to integrate this unexpected awareness into daily life, I encountered and created significant suffering—for myself and others. The intensity of my experience produced a widening gap between what I now held as Truth and what I knew to be illusion. The Love and unity I felt contrasted sharply with the struggles and disconnections inherent in human existence. I fought to get back what I believed I'd lost; to achieve an effortless state of Enlightenment or Sahaja from where there would be no returning to Maia, the illusion.

The more I fought, the more I became trapped once more in the shadow side of my earthly existence, all the while avoiding the discomfort of unresolved emotions, attachments, and a personal history steeped in trauma and loss. The very Love that had illuminated my being now exposed my shortcomings. And I did not like the person I was.

In my eagerness to regain my otherworldly treasure, I failed to acknowledge the pain I was causing to those around me. Attempts to express the bliss of my experience overshadowed others' feelings, creating misunderstandings and emotional distance. My awareness of soul contracts led me to neglect the immediate needs of those I cared for, and even fueled the sort of exploitative behavior that a forsaken shadow will always create. Ultimately, I ended up inflicting great suffering on another, with its ripple casting heartache over many more.

I did not accept it at the time, but my own suffering in the aftermath of this awakening became a teacher in its own right. It stripped away the idealization of spiritual enlightenment, forcing me to ground more deeply into an illusion that I had come to detest. It forced me to address my shortcomings, finally acknowledge my shadow, and learn to love all my unlovely parts. It pressed me to acquire self-compassion so that I could *be* compassionate—and empathetic and sensitive—to others. It tasked me to become more *fully* human.

Through this realization, I now strive to approach others with greater awareness, recognizing that each soul's journey is interwoven with my own. In this moment and every moment, life is a profound exploration of connection, purpose, and a Love that is guided through the mostly unconscious recognition that we are all god aspects of the same divine Consciousness; whirlpools each, but entangled together in a seamless ocean.

Awakening is not an individual journey, but one that we do together. Our suffering is an opportunity for deeper connection and healing, allowing us to embrace the full experience of embodiment as we navigate the sacred, shared journey of our souls. As I reflect on my actions, misdeeds, and all that makes me ugly, I begin to understand that real growth comes not only from transcending suffering, but also from embracing it. And so I come to appreciate that Love and suffering coexist as essential elements, each providing depth and richness to the experience of being alive.

But the greatest of these is Love.

"Silence is the language of God, all else is poor translation."

— Rūmī

Stay Connected!

As you reach the end of this book, take a moment to acknowledge the profound healing journey you have embarked upon. Through curiously exploring your symptoms, feelings, thoughts, and life experiences, you are weaving together the intricate drivers of your GERD. This exploration is not merely a means of understanding your disease; it is a foundational step toward uncovering personal meaning, healing and authentic empowerment.

By reflecting on the unity of factors in your story that come together to produce personal meaning, you are cultivating awareness of your unique emotional, psychological and physical landscape. You are gaining the tools to recognize limiting beliefs, understand the burden of your old narrative, and create an alternative, nourishing inner dialog of curiosity, openness, and compassion.

Healing is not a destination, but a continuously unfolding journey into the depths of self-awareness. As you integrate each new insight, remember that every step you take contributes to a broader understanding of your wholeperson. Embrace this unitary approach as it nurtures your well-being.

Your story matters, and sharing it can inspire yours and others' healing. Together, let's create a community that embraces the diversity of chronic illnesses and prioritizes a MindBody or meaning-based story approach to emotional, psychological and physical well-being. Thank you for joining me on this transformative journey. Your healing and empowerment is yours to unfold.

If you'd like to get in touch for any reason, please check out the Contact page on my website: **https://howardchristian.com/contact**

Your Home Remedy for Acid Reflux Disease

Free Companion Resources

Enhance your journey with *Your Home Remedy for Acid Reflux Disease: Live, Eat and Heal Abundantly* by unlocking a treasure trove of FREE Companion Resources. Dive into symptom-mood charts, exclusive audio exercises, and a transformative MindBody workbook designed to accelerate your healing from acid reflux disease/GERD. And this is just the beginning—stay tuned for more bonus content coming your way!

Don't wait—visit the link below to gain instant access and enhance your journey to wellness today!

HOWARDCHRISTIAN.COM/READER-COMPANION-RESOURCES

Live, Eat and Heal Abundantly

Printed in Great Britain
by Amazon